Let's Talk Radiation Therapy

An Insider's Guide for Patients Facing the Anxiety, Process, & Side Effects of This Cancer Treatment

by

Margeaux Gregory, R.T.(T)

Distribution by Bublish

Editing by Bublish

Published by Radiation Therapy Explained LLC

ISBN: 9781647048129 (eBook)

ISBN: 9781647048105 (paperback)

ISBN: 9781647048112 (hardcover)

Cover design and format: We Are Almanac LLC

Front cover photography: Alisha Maria Photography

Dedicated to newly diagnosed cancer patients and inspired by the outcome of their success.

Contents

Preface

Dear Reader,

Thank you so much for trusting me in this vulnerable time of your life. I am so honored you have chosen to be here. I've worked on the front lines of radiation oncology for over fifteen years, delivering thousands of external beam radiation treatments to cancer patients from all walks of life, circumstances, ages, and religions. To be trusted so intimately with a cancer patient's care is not a responsibility I take lightly. I've made it my mission to bring peace through understanding to every patient I've encountered. I deeply believe in the importance of helping people grasp *why* we are doing what we are doing and how this contributes to them receiving the best care possible. Helping people discover their own courage using relevant knowledge as they navigate this process is what feeds my soul in this work.

My comfort level counseling numerous family members and friends with their cancer diagnoses outside of the clinic led me to explore being able to reach even more people with the type of advice I found myself giving. Upon each person's diagnosis, I would offer to discuss their circumstances with them, helping answer technical and logistical questions, and emotional ones as well. It became quite clear to me how the uncertainty surrounding their experiences left them on unsteady ground mentally. Information and conversation that came relatively easily to me seemed to genuinely help them, and I was more than happy to alleviate some of their anxieties surrounding their impending treatment. I could hear the relief in their voices after our conversations, and I felt proud to be of help outside of the clinic walls. I found that by simply explaining these topics a few steps further, I could help them begin to rebuild their peace of mind. Sharing knowledge with them that supported their experiences gave them strength, as it uncovered a small portion of this new "unknown." I soon realized there was a need to address the conversation surrounding receiving radiation treatment differently, because somewhere along the line, vital information that could support peace of mind was falling through the cracks.

Over the years, I've noticed many patients feeling overwhelmed, grasping for answers, and being confused by the scattered gathering of information in the time immediately after their confirmed cancer diagnoses. It became apparent to me that many people began this experience the same way: feeling overwhelmed by the magnitude of information out there and not being able to make sense of what steps they should anticipate next. Information currently accessible to patients seems to only scratch the surface in helping them face the cancer treatment process. This book aims to bridge that gap and help newly diagnosed cancer patients feel more in control and appropriately informed by providing clarity about the process leading up to choosing a modality as well as what they can expect if they've chosen to pursue radiation treatment.

Through my experience, I have learned that caring for cancer patients is truly multifaceted. While I recognize that it is critically important to provide appropriate treatment physically, it is impossible to ignore the weight of the emotional complexities linked to this type of life-changing diagnosis.

Most of this book is designed to provide you, the reader, with technical information about the treatment process; however, as I was writing, I couldn't deny how important it felt to me to nurture the emotional aspect of the process as well. It felt natural for me to present all this information to you in the same way I would for a loved one—as if you were joining me for a walk on the beach so we could talk all about it.

At the end of each chapter, I present you with the opportunity to pause our walk and digest the information you've just read. The serenity of the beach has always provided me with a place where my head and heart heal; I hope you will also find that serenity and healing on our walk through this book.

I want to give you, my reader, the opportunity to find real answers, all in one place, that will help uncover the intricacies of the radiation treatment process and give you the courage to take your next steps. I hope that my expertise will give you strength so you can feel much more in control, significantly more prepared, and in the know. Having a bit more knowledge will help you approach this whole process with solid footing and allow you to assemble a strategy to proceed with your radiation treatment—one that encourages inner strength and peace of mind. That sounds like a much better place to start from than uncertainty and confusion, and it's a starting point I'm honored to guide you toward. I'm eager to help you feel better about embarking on this process, so let's get started.

With love and gratitude,

Margeaux

Introduction

Receiving a cancer diagnosis can be unsettling at best. Trying to manage your erupting fears of uncertainty for what lies ahead while attempting to maintain a clear head to process the next steps can be emotionally upending, to say the least. With the hurried scheduling of new medical appointments and managing the sometimes differing opinions for treatment, it's difficult not to feel overly stressed and in cancer's control—not to mention the infringement on your personal space after intimate conversations surrounding your body, invasive physical exams, and medical imaging quickly become commonplace. It can be so easy to feel overwhelmed by everything you don't know.

With the stakes so high and many options for treatment, proceeding with a clear head can feel elusive as you grapple with these circumstances. Arriving at the first few appointments unsure of what to expect or what questions to ask can bring those feelings of dread and vulnerability right to the surface. I've witnessed the full spectrum of emotions from people who are just beginning their cancer treatment course, and I need you to know that you are not alone in this struggle.

Over the course of my career, I've helped thousands of people push past their anxieties and fears about receiving radiation treatment by imparting my knowledge about what they can expect from their upcoming encounters in the radiation oncology department. I'm passionate about guiding people through their radiation experiences by helping them understand, in detail, what will be happening at their appointments. Furthermore, I make it my goal to help them understand the *reasons* behind our actions and requests. I've seen how powerful this type of explanation can be in order to help people ground their thoughts and feel more in control. Creating this environment allows people to feel more prepared, encouraging a much calmer and controlled energy and placing them in a better headspace to participate in decisions surrounding their care.

I know that having the right information can be integral in creating a positive shift in your mental health while going through cancer treatment, and I'm eager to bring you that peace of mind within these pages. Before you learn about the specifics of radiation therapy, I also believe it will be very helpful for you to understand a little bit about the different health care providers (HCPs) involved in the world of oncology and the types of treatment each of them offers. These HCPs include doctors, physicians, physician assistants, social workers, radiation therapists, medical oncologists, nurses, nurse practitioners, medical assistants, and more. By gaining a general understanding about what defines each of their specialties, you will also grasp how they work together as a team to provide comprehensive cancer care. Ultimately, being able to differentiate between the basic responsibilities of each HCP will help you alleviate significant confusion right from the start. Your familiarity with this new information will undoubtedly help you feel more prepared by providing some structure, allowing you to arrive at your appointments less unnerved and feeling more *ready*.

Once you've developed an overarching understanding of oncology in general, you will have a clearer idea of the role of radiation therapy. In this book, you can expect to learn *why* and *how* radiation can be a very effective way to treat cancer, what to anticipate from your treatment team, and what getting radiation treatment can look like. I will explain our sometimes complicated processes in a manner that is easy to digest. You will discover detailed information that is key to understanding our methodology as clinicians and how this directly corresponds to your experience as a patient. You will learn about our goals when designing and implementing your highly individualized radiation treatment plan and how this relates to your cancer care. I will also review the stringent protocols in place that keep you safe in our treatment room. For the times when receiving radiation treatments can become particularly challenging, I will show you how to use your new understanding of radiation science to dispel self-sabotaging thoughts and continue through to successful completion of your radiation treatment. I have extensive experience coaching others just like you through each and every radiation treatment, and I'm eager to expand my outreach beyond the clinic walls to the pages of this book.

Fortunately, we live in a time when our understanding of cancer's intricacies and the options for treatment are so much more effective than in years past. The medical community's understanding of cancer behaviors has advanced leaps and bounds and continues to do so each day with the offering of highly tailored treatments and advancements in technology. The way we used to think dismally about a cancer diagnosis in years past is now challenged by the comprehensive understanding of this disease and the different angles by which we can successfully treat, attack, and destroy the function of cancer cells in the body.

I believe this book will help you work toward your own goal of advocating and participating in healing for yourself. After reading it, you should feel significantly less intimidated and far more prepared to navigate your own next steps. So let's get you ready to learn about radiation therapy in a different light. I'm not about approaching the discussion surrounding cancer treatment with a shy or somber attitude; in fact, I feel quite the opposite. I recognize that this topic can be heavy, but our conversation doesn't have to be. I am confident that your having this knowledge can help you approach treatment with self-generated strength and an overall sense of readiness. By walking right through your fears, you will learn to be a better advocate for yourself throughout this radiation treatment process.

I want to make sure my message is loud and clear: I need you to believe that you can get through this, because I've seen it firsthand *thousands* of times. Just because you're up against this diagnosis doesn't mean your only choice is to sink into submissiveness and hand over the reins to this disease. This book will show you how to take charge and get what you need—medically, emotionally, and educationally. It will prime you to move forward and select a treatment and a team that feels intentional, reassuring, and helpful for you specifically.

It can be so frustrating to feel as though so much is out of your control when you have health challenges. It may seem as if there's nothing you can do about it. But there *is* something you can do about it. You can educate yourself and prepare yourself, and by reading this book, you're doing just that! I am just one piece of this support, but I can't encourage you enough to advocate for yourself at this time. After finishing this book, you will be able to trust that you have this knowledge, understand this process, and can proceed through treatment. I know you have the grit and courage, because you're reading these words! So please allow me to give you information that will inspire you to move forward confidently.

I'm ready to help you find your footing and confidence by giving you the tools for self-empowerment during this trying time. Anxiety thrives on uncertainties. Let's challenge that by getting you to feel certain that you understand the process, can manage your anxiety, and can approach this time in your life with self-belief and self-generated strength. I can't make your treatment easier for you, but I *can* make you smarter about it. With these smarts comes strength, and with strength comes confidence. Let's help you *feel prepared*. Let's help you *get ready*.

I invite you to kick off your shoes, take a deep breath, and meet me at the beach. Without further ado, please walk the shoreline with me. Let's talk radiation therapy.

1

Pre-appointment Madness
of the Unknown

How to Take Back Control, Choose a Treatment,
Find the Right Team of Doctors, and Get in the Know

It's an understatement to say the window of time right after a cancer diagnosis and before treatment begins is a whirlwind. Being suddenly thrown into the world of oncology uninformed can feel overwhelming, especially when the stakes are so high. With an abundance of information available, how do you even know where to start? At a minimum, you've probably asked yourself, *What treatment do I need? What physicians do I need to see? What are the basics surrounding the different treatment options, and which is right for me?* Breaking down this process into digestible information for a better understanding can be integral to slowing the inundation of thoughts and establishing your footing. Being properly informed will encourage a sense of calm as your thoughts become somewhat collected. Now, when you meet with the experts, you'll feel prepared and ready to discuss your best options for treatment. Get ready to push fear aside, dispel confusion, and shed some light on this process.

Let's start building this knowledge by introducing you to the oncology team from a broader perspective. Once you understand the basic oncology dynamics, you'll be able to approach your consultations with a better comprehension of each provider's responsibilities, as well as how they all work together. Even if you approach your consultations with only this basic information, you will undoubtedly feel more prepared and self-assured than if you went into your appointments without any preparation. You're giving yourself the gift of starting this process from a place of readiness. This energy will foster productive discussions, allowing you to choose a treatment plan that you can feel great about and that aligns with your goals, head, and heart.

Who are the main oncology physicians, and what do they do?

Radiation Oncologist: The physician who will be constructing and directing your radiation treatment. They will work closely in collaboration with surgical and medical oncologists to design a comprehensive cancer treatment plan for you, focusing specifically on your radiation treatment. They will decide the total and daily radiation dose you'll receive, and how many treatments you'll have. (This is the physician I work for directly.)

Medical Oncologist: The physician who is responsible for directing and designing your chemotherapy, immunotherapy, and other drug therapy treatments. They will work closely with your radiation oncologist if it is decided that you will have systemic drug or chemotherapy treatments in addition to the radiation therapy treatment.

Surgical Oncologist: A surgeon who specializes in oncology. Typically, the techniques, processes, and skill sets are more specialized than that of a general surgeon. They will work closely with the radiation oncologist to help understand where the cancer is in your body. Additionally, if any fragment of tumor was unable to be removed, they would relay this to your radiation oncologist so it can be included in the area for radiation treatment.

What can I do to prepare for the first meeting with my oncology physicians?

One of the first things you can do is think about what your goals are for your cancer treatment. This may seem like a ridiculous point, as most people's goal is to get rid of this cancer yesterday; however, different circumstances in life will present different desires and expectations from treatment. Allow me to explain. Someone in their late eighties might choose treatment that isn't as aggressive and would allow them to simply be a little more comfortable for a few more years. Alternatively, someone in their early thirties might choose to be very aggressive with their treatment, opting for multiple angles of treatment such as chemo, radiation, and surgery, as they desire and expect to be on this earth for many more years. I encourage you to show up to your meetings with the physicians knowing your goals for treatment so your conversations can be more constructive and get you closer to the exact answers you're seeking.

Who are the people working behind the scenes involved in the details of my diagnosis?

Although you will not likely meet these people, they serve as an integral support team for your physicians in helping learn vitally important information about *your* cancer cells. The fact that you even have a specific diagnosis comes from the knowledge these scientists provide. These team members study the cells from your biopsy to help understand the nuances of the cancer in your body. The information they provide will help your providers narrow down the most effective options for treatment.

Pathologist: A board-certified member of the team who studies fluids, cells, and tissues taken from your biopsy. They support your physicians in determining exactly what cell mutations are present in your type of cancer and will determine your official cancer diagnosis.

Microbiologist: A member of the team who is responsible for studying cells and cell behavior. They study the microbiome, cell mutations, and immune interactions of your cells to help understand which treatments will be most effective and safe for you and your cancer, specifically.

Immunologist: A member of the team who is board certified and responsible for studying how your body's own natural immune system response affects the cancer cells in your body. By understanding the biological connection between your immune system and your cancer, the immunologist provides your oncology team with information that can help determine which drug treatments will be most effective in using your own immune system to help fight your cancer.

Genetic Counselor: Speaking in the world of oncology specifically, this team member will meet with you to review the results that the geneticist, pathologist, and biologist provide. They will be able to help you understand if there is a hereditary link in your genes for your cancer that could be passed down from, or to, your blood relatives. Essentially, this type of information could be very useful if your parents had cancer, you developed the same cancer, and you're concerned about your children being at risk for this same cancer. I like to say that genetic testing essentially provides you with an awareness of any genetically inherited risk of cancer. This type of testing is not available for *every* type of cancer, but if you're curious or interested, you can certainly ask your radiation oncologist if this type of testing is an option for you.

Personal Story:

As I've mentioned previously, I've had a lot of experience coaching friends and family outside of the clinic who have been diagnosed with cancer. Unfortunately, one of those people was my mother. She was diagnosed with breast cancer a few years back. Luckily for us, she had a great understanding of this process and the treatment options available to her (along with a great attitude!), as she works in radiation oncology as a medical dosimetrist. (You'll learn more about the role of

this professional in the radiation oncology department in chapter 3.)
As part of her oncologic workup at the time of diagnosis, she opted for
genetic testing. It felt important for her to know if she carried a genetic
mutation that could put her children at risk for this same type of can-
cer. Fortunately, her results revealed that there was no genetic mutation
for breast cancer that she carried hereditarily that could be passed on
to her children. Having concrete information about her own truth,
pertinent to her own health specifically, is one piece of this puzzle that
has provided her with significant peace of mind.

Why am I being sent for imaging/blood work/additional appointments ahead of my meetings with the physicians?

There are a few things your physician might ask of you in preparation for your consultations. This information will help them narrow down and determine the optimal treatment options for *you specifically*. Most commonly, if you haven't already done so, the physicians might request that you get some diagnostic imaging scans done. These might include a PET (Positron Emission Tomography) scan, an MRI (Magnetic Resonance Imaging), a CT (Computed Tomography) scan, ultrasound, and more. It can be a little frustrating to have additional appointments before the ball even gets rolling, but I promise you that the information these scans provide will give your physicians the clarity and knowledge to help them determine your best options for treatment.

These scans help them understand exactly *where* the cancer is located in your body and *what* the predictable behavior is for your type of cancer. Identifying the exact areas where disease is present in your body is crucial in designing an effective and complex cancer treatment. I strongly implore you to follow through with any appointments they've requested, as it will only support your physicians in precisely choosing accurate, safe, and effective treatment specific to you.

What are the different scans I might expect, and what are they used for?

PET Scan: A diagnostic medical imaging scan that uses an injectable radioactive chemical (called a *radiotracer*) to visualize areas in the body where there is increased cellular activity. This type of scan is useful for determining where microscopic disease could be present in your body.

MRI: A diagnostic medical imaging scan that does not use radiation; rather, it uses a combination of radio waves and magnetic fields to create detailed images. This type of imaging is useful for seeing delineation among soft tissues within the body.

CT Scan: A medical imaging technique that produces three-dimensional images of the inside of the body. Sometimes contrast will be used for this diagnostic scan. Contrast can be administered orally (by mouth) or intravenous injection (by vein), or not at all. This decision is at the discretion of the physician who ordered the scan. If contrast is injected, it is used to highlight the features of the blood vessels clearly. If contrast is swallowed by mouth, it will display the features of the digestive tract.

Ultrasound: A noninvasive diagnostic imaging technique that creates images by using sound waves. This type of imaging can be helpful for visualizing lymph nodes or other structures that might be close to the skin's surface. There is no radiographic exposure involved.

How do I find the treatment that is right for me?

I can certainly understand why you would scour the Internet in the hopes of finding information that will reveal the perfect treatment for your cancer. But although research is great for gathering basic information about your cancer and the treatment options available, I would caution you not to concretely decide on a specific type of treatment because of what you read online. Too many times, I've seen patients push to receive a specific type of treatment that was not clinically appropriate for them.

They were reluctant to be convinced otherwise because that was the conclusion they'd arrived at from their own research. They were not in a headspace to *listen and learn* why that option might not be the most appropriate choice for them, and the disconnect between their research and the team's explanation left them feeling disappointed, defeated, and confused before everything had even gotten started. So, how *can* you participate in finding the best treatment for yourself?

It is inevitable that you'll search the Internet for information about your type of cancer—and rightfully so. While having accurate baseline information about your cancer and the treatments available is important, your best bet is to have a general idea of options available for treatment but be ready to get the most accurate answers from your oncology physicians. It's highly unlikely that you'll have a better understanding of the best treatment options for you than your treatment team will. It's best to view these professionals as your personal set of encyclopedias for the latest and greatest treatments available.

I want to help you manage your expectations before you go to the clinic, because handling the disappointment of not having it go exactly as you believed it would can be emotionally challenging at an already sensitive time. Please find peace in knowing that the research is being done for you, and that it is *not* your responsibility to navigate these intricacies and choose the perfect treatment. Try not to get tunnel vision in finding the perfect treatment. Rather, focus your research on two things: the basic options available for your type of cancer and selecting an oncology team you trust.

Finding the Best Treatment for Your Cancer and Why the Answer Is Not Simple

Finding a "blanket cure" for cancer as a disease is challenging because there are many unique genetic mutations of cancer cells. Rarely are any two lifestyles, circumstances, stages, levels of baseline health, or patients alike. Also, there are many combinations for treatment options and choices these days that are ever-changing even as this book goes to print—which can feel like a blessing and a curse when you're first dipping your toes in the water surrounding this diagnosis and trying to tackle it alone.

Connie, one of my former coworkers and a radiation therapist herself, described it best when she recounted what a radiation oncologist she once worked for said about choosing the appropriate treatment for his patients. He told her, "To best treat cancer with a curative intent, you must study cancer and its treatments as an art, really." I couldn't have said it better myself! You should feel confident in knowing that behind the scenes, cancer is being studied and researched to understand the complexities, nuances, and minutiae surrounding the cells and their behaviors. Your oncology providers are consistently developing and discussing new research and protocols. They collaborate on a community, national, and international level by sharing new techniques, technologies, and breakthroughs.

When I first started working at a hospital world renowned for its innovation, research, and collaboration, even I was astounded by the constant dedication to improvements, breakthroughs, and continual developments in cancer care. Treatments are improving and evolving, and, therefore, it is unreasonable—and frankly inappropriate—to expect patients to have the most up-to-date information readily accessible on the Internet.

Did you know that even though you might have the same type of cancer as someone else—breast cancer, for example—that even within that type of cancer there are multiple subtypes of different cell mutations that can be present, each requiring different protocols and treatments? So, just because you know someone who had breast cancer and got chemo, that doesn't necessarily mean *you* should also receive chemo because you have breast cancer.

Each cancer diagnosis comes with its own set of intricacies personal to you, which is why the treatment should be specifically tailored to you, and why it's crucial that your research not be focused solely on treatments but rather on finding a team of professionals you can trust.

Guidance for Finding the Right Oncology Team

Instead of searching for the "perfect treatment" for your cancer, I implore you to focus your research efforts on finding physicians who have previous experience in treating the type of cancer you have. If you have a common type of cancer, it could be relatively easy to find oncologists within a reasonable traveling distance. If your cancer is rare or located in an anatomically intricate area of your body, you might find that you need to travel to receive safe and appropriate treatment. With so many brilliant and dedicated oncology physicians out there, how do you know that you've picked the right one?

I can't stress enough how important it is to find an oncology team you feel like you can trust. Choosing your treatment team is a very personal decision and one that *you*, as the person receiving treatment, need to be comfortable with.

Some people find comfort in older physicians due to their years of experience practicing medicine. Others find comfort in younger physicians who they feel might have more information and cutting-edge attitudes. Some people don't want to endure the hassle of longer travel and prefer to receive treatment locally, while others know immediately that they only want care from a certain hospital and will travel or do whatever it takes to receive care at that institution. Choosing your physician is a personal task and should really be focused on the wishes and goals of the individual receiving treatment.

You will know when you've met the right physician for you when you feel an overarching sense of relief that stems from *trust*. You should feel heard, not rushed or dismissed, and as if you're in the hands of someone who knows what they're talking about. They should have confident answers to your questions, even if they might not be answers you want to hear. You should be able to address your concerns and fears and ask them anything without feeling judged. They should have your goals in mind and offer you treatment that supports those aims. You should feel relieved to have them direct your care because you trust they will do right by you. The pressure of choosing the perfect treatment now falls on *their* shoulders, right where it should be. It is their job to develop the details and understand your best options so you can receive the best possible treatment.

You should be able to tell your physician exactly what you're afraid of regarding your treatment so they can tailor their solutions with this in mind. It also allows them to be as honest as possible with you so you can understand the expectations of this treatment, within reason. Keeping this in mind, when you walk out of that office after your meeting, you should feel like you can take the deepest, most stress-relieving breath you've taken in weeks. Leave the pressure and stress of designing your treatment to the physician you trust. You'll know you've found the right one for you when you feel heard and are being confidently guided in their care.

What if my family or loved ones do not agree with my choice for treatment or my treatment team?

It's great to have support from family or loved ones during this process, but sometimes they might not agree with your choices. Truthfully, it is not up to *them* how *you* handle *your* diagnosis. When you lie down at night, *you* are the only one dealing with the thoughts in your head. I encourage you to be the director of your own peace. Acknowledge what is important to you, and own it. Although there is certainly room for family and friends to have their own feelings about your diagnosis and be affected in their own way, their body is different from yours, and sometimes your choices might be different too. Ultimately, I need you to know that this choice is yours. If you are at peace with your choice in treatment, your family and loved ones will feel that from you and likely get behind your decision, even if they might have chosen differently.

How do I know if I should get a second opinion?

If you meet with an oncologist and you feel that they're dismissive of your goals or concerns, they have an abrasive bedside manner, or you just aren't getting a great feeling surrounding their care, it's not a bad idea to get a second opinion. Remember, you should feel that your physicians are relieving stress from you, not contributing to it. Make sure you don't wait too long to seek additional consultation, as taking care of the cancer as early as possible is single-handedly one of the most advantageous things you can do to eradicate the disease for good. Your team should be providing you with information and guiding you in your decisions so you can choose a treatment you feel great about—*together*. You can ask your physician how long the "grace period" is before you need to decide about your treatment. They will let you know accurate timelines based on your current circumstances.

My physicians are all at different hospitals. Is this okay?

Finding a center where all your care can be done in the same hospital or buildings can make your experience a little more seamless and a little bit less stressful; however, this is certainly not necessary in order to receive excellent care. When all the departments have established lines of communication already in place, this can be very helpful with coordinating appointments and your care.

If you're receiving care at a few different hospitals, it will be very helpful to be organized and proactive right from the start. First, establish one secure place to keep all medical contact information. Ensure it's readily available to you, either on your phone or in a notebook. Before ending your appointment with a provider (and while you're still in the room together), gather their contact information. Ask them for their preferred method of communication if you were to be asked by another health care provider. Also, it's a simple thing to overlook, but write down what type of care this physician is providing (what they are responsible for) and their title. Avoid any confusion for yourself, and make sure your notes are legible and easy for you to understand. When you have this information organized and effortlessly at your fingertips, you will be able to easily bridge any communication gaps confidently and instantly. You will be setting up your future self for success by organizing this information from the beginning. Additionally, it can be helpful to bring a friend or family member with you to help record or recall information.

Let's take a moment and pause our walk at the shoreline.

Give yourself some time to digest this new information.

Inhale the fresh air as you recognize how proud you feel for pushing past your nerves and taking these first steps. You're beginning to understand a little bit more about how you desire to move forward, and it feels good to have gained some clarity amid this initial chaos.

Exhale the fear and anxiety, which does not serve you.

Take as much time with this breathwork as you like.

Take in the fresh smell of the ocean, and feel the gritty sand under your toes, the sun on your face, and me by your side. You feel present in this moment as we look out over the ocean in admiration of what Mother Nature has created—the marine life, the coral, the sand, the rocks—all existing in a world mostly known only to them.

Now, among all the wonder that Mother Nature has created in these waters, a new addition of a seemingly out-of-place object appears. It's a glass bottle, newly broken, its separate pieces now in disarray as they slowly meander toward the ocean floor.

When you're feeling ready to learn more, let's walk.

2

Radiation Therapy, Chemotherapy, Surgery, and Other Drug Therapies

What's the Difference?

There are several combinations for tailoring a highly effective, safe, and complex cancer treatment. Our understanding of cancer's behavior and the options for treatment have become so much more effective and advanced than in years past. You cannot imagine how many people are dedicated behind the scenes to the study of these diseases and the continual development of new and effective treatments—it's incredible! Even in the fifteen-plus years I've worked in this field, I've seen significant advancements in the technologies and the treatments offered. Because of the ever-advancing nature of effective treatments, it's best to have a discussion with your oncology team to determine the best combinations and options for you.

Discussions you might have with your oncology team may focus on a singular therapy or a combination of therapies—and how these all can align with your goals for treatment. There are multiple options to curate the perfect treatment for you. Don't let this fact overwhelm you, but rather, let it bring you comfort. Utilizing your oncology experts to help choose an effective treatment that aligns with your goals has never been more attainable than it is today.

Radiation Therapy

Radiation therapy refers to the therapeutic use of a high dose of radiation to treat and kill cancer cells. This kind of cancer treatment is *localized*—meaning it does not go all through your body and will only be delivered to an exact, pinpointed location. Sometimes radiation therapy can be used by itself, and sometimes it will be used in combination with other types of cancer treatment therapies. There can be various combinations, and the best choice will be determined by your specific circumstances: how big the tumor is, where it is in your body, the type of cancer you have, and so on. You will rely on your cancer specialists to provide you with their best recommendation for highly effective treatment.

Surgery

Surgery is also a localized treatment. It may be one of the first steps of your cancer treatment but not always. Surgery can be a great place to start, as it can physically remove the cancer in your body. It can remove the tumor and ultimately the entirety of the cancer if you're lucky, resulting in this being the only cancer treatment you might need.

Sometimes we can use surgery to *debulk* the tumor. This means the entirety of the tumor cannot be removed with surgery, but the surgeon will be able to significantly decrease its size within your body. This type of surgery is an option if your tumor is located near critical or sensitive structures in the body, and the surgeon is unable to safely remove all of it without affecting other systems.

Chemotherapy

Chemotherapy is the use of drugs to kill microscopic cancer disease throughout your body. Treatments administered to the whole body as opposed to a localized area are referred to as *systemic*. This type of treatment is great if your physicians are concerned about microscopic disease potentially present in other areas of the body not located directly where the tumor is present.

Hormone Therapy, Immunotherapy, and Other Drug Therapies

There are new treatments emerging to aid the oncology community in fighting cancer as a disease, and drug therapies are certainly one of them. As I've mentioned a few times before, researchers are continually working to advance cancer therapies. Physician investigators, scientists, and researchers are finding new ways to treat cancer not only with surgery, radiation, and chemo but also with novel approaches such as cutting off the cancer's food source. Brilliant, right? This type of hormone therapy can work for certain cancers that use your hormones as a food source, the premise being that if we can alter, diminish, or slow down cancer's food source, we can slow or stop the growth of that cancer.

Immunotherapy is a type of drug treatment that can boost or aid your body's own immune system as another option for cancer treatment. Using the understanding of our body's natural immune response, scientists and researchers are now developing ways to assist the body's own immune system in its attack against cancer cells. Whether it's using drugs to stimulate a stronger immune response, assisting our own immune cells by helping them identify cancer cells, or using laboratory science to aid our body's own fight, these drug therapies offer another approach for cancer treatment.

There is quite a bit of research surrounding these new treatment types, but we learn more and more each day about which patients will benefit from immunotherapy and how best to administer the treatment. Although these treatments are not an effective option for everyone, you can ask your clinicians if any of these drug therapies may be an option for you.

Radiation Therapy and Surgery

There are a few ways in which radiation therapy can work together with surgery. The size and location of the tumor will affect the order of surgery and radiation. If the tumor is quite large, we can sometimes irradiate first to potentially shrink the size of it a little before surgery.

Sometimes surgery will be done first to remove as much of the tumor as possible, then radiation will follow the surgery. If there is the concern that residual tumor might be present after surgery (called *positive margins*), it's possible you could have radiation to ensure eradication of the disease. Radiation works great with surgery as a localized treatment combination that can be delivered directly to the area where the tumor was extracted and to any residual microscopic tumor potentially left behind in that same area.

Radiation Therapy and Chemotherapy

It's quite common for radiation therapy and chemotherapy to be used in conjunction. Since chemo is a systemic treatment and radiation is a localized treatment, this combination is quite comprehensive and one we see often. The order in which radiation and chemotherapy are delivered can vary. Sometimes you can receive a few rounds of chemotherapy and then radiation. Alternatively, radiation can be delivered first, with chemotherapy to follow. It's also possible for radiation and chemotherapy to be delivered at the same time. In this instance, chemotherapy acts as a *radiosensitizer*. This means that chemotherapy can enhance the effectiveness of radiation treatment. As I've mentioned before, there are multiple combinations for cancer treatment success, and the determination of which is best depends on each person's individual circumstances.

Radiation Therapy and Other Drug Therapies

Radiation can be given independently or in combination with other drug therapies. Sometimes you might have separate *cycles*, when you receive your course of radiation, then continue treatment with a drug therapy. Also, radiation and your drug therapy can be given at the same time, or drug therapy can precede radiation. Again, there are multiple combinations that will best be decided by your oncology experts.

***

Let's take a moment and pause our walk at the shoreline.

Stand with me at the shoreline as you take a moment to absorb this new information.

Inhale the fresh air as you acknowledge how great it feels to be actively pursuing the perfect treatment combination. You're slowly starting to feel moments of clarity, and you feel some relief from your stress.

Exhale the anxiety that does not serve you.

As we stand here admiring the serenity of the ocean, I find my mind wandering back to that glass bottle. Its pieces that were once a unified whole now lie on the ocean floor. I begin to wonder what impact the bottle encountered—an impact so powerful that it created change of this magnitude. What stood so solidly for so long in the same form is now undeniably different.

Take the time you need here, and just breathe.

When you're feeling ready, let's continue our walk.

3

Meet the Radiation Oncology Staff

Learn Who Can Get Your Needs Met and What to
Expect at Your Consultation

I'd like to start with a brief introduction to some important staff members within the radiation oncology department who will be involved, both directly and indirectly, with your care. Some of these people, like your radiation therapists, you will interact with each day. Some of these people you will likely not meet, as their involvement is a little bit more behind the scenes, but they still play an integral role in getting you treated effectively, safely, and efficiently. You'll hear me reference these different HCPs and their roles as you explore the information ahead.

Staff you will frequently encounter throughout
your radiation treatment:

Radiation Oncologist: This is your radiation physician. You will meet with them at your consultation to discuss radiation therapy and how it could be beneficial for you. They decide the total amount of radiation you'll receive, how many treatments it will take to deliver the total prescribed dose, and what dose you'll receive daily. Once you've started treatment, you'll see them for weekly check-ins alongside your radiation nurse. This weekly check-in is often referred to as an *on-treatment visit* (OTV) or *weekly treatment management* (WTM).

<u>Radiation Nurse:</u> This nurse works specifically with your radiation oncologist. They will help you manage your side effects and will be a great liaison between you and other HCPs for any questions or concerns. You will see them for your weekly check-ins and/or on an as-needed basis.

<u>Radiation Therapist:</u> (My role on the oncology team!) You will see this team member every day, as they are responsible for delivering the radiation treatments. They are a great resource for treatment questions, so don't be afraid to ask them about whatever is on your mind. If they can't answer your question, they will know exactly which team member you should speak with to get some answers.

Additional staff in radiation oncology:

<u>Physician's Assistant (PA):</u> This is a highly trained and board-certified member of the team who will support the duties of your radiation oncologist. They can be involved in all aspects of your care, including evaluation and caring for patients who are undergoing radiation treatment.

<u>Nurse Practitioner (NP):</u> This is an advanced practice registered nurse who has additional education and board certification beyond that of a registered nurse. They work closely in collaboration with radiation oncologists as a provider, caring for patients actively receiving treatment, as well as patients who have finished treatment. You can also encounter this professional in cancer prevention, screening, research, and surgery.

<u>Medical Assistant (MA):</u> An MA working in radiation oncology would be responsible for supporting the physicians and nurses in the department. They would likely be the member of the team to take your vitals, record your general health history, collect specimens, and so on.

<u>Front Desk Administrative Staff:</u> These staff members will be responsible for checking you in at the front desk for your treatment each day. Also, they will most likely be able to guide you with insurance questions or scheduling diagnostic imaging appointments, if that has been requested by your physician.

Your treatment team behind the scenes:

Medical Physicist: This is a board-certified member of the team responsible for the maintenance, upkeep, and operation of the linear accelerator (the machine that delivers the radiation treatments) and CT simulator in the department. They oversee the radiation treatment planning and quality assurance for the linear accelerator as well as individualized treatment plans.

Medical Dosimetrist: This member of the team is board certified and highly trained to understand how different body tissues tolerate radiation. They will develop and design the optimal radiation treatment plan for you, your body, and your cancer specifically, based on the directives from the radiation oncologist.

Who are some additional (optional) people I could meet with if I'm curious about gaining more information or facing some challenges?

Social Worker: This member of the team is a phenomenal resource for social and emotional support. You can meet with them on an as-needed basis if you'd like someone to talk to or just want someone to listen. They can provide you with contact information and inform you about support groups for patients like yourself, so you can create a community of care that feels custom designed to you.

Support Group: Finding people who are facing the same health challenges as you can provide a surprising amount of support for you while you're going through treatment—and even after you've completed it. Being with those who can understand and relate to what you're going through can be more encouraging and comforting than you might initially think. Some patients have found success with online community support (with people who share a similar diagnosis), and some patients attend support groups that are run in their radiation department. It is entirely up to you what type of support you prefer, but I would implore you to find someone you feel like you can talk to openly and honestly. Having a trusted outlet for conversation is important for healing and for supporting your mental health.

<u>Nutritionist:</u> This member of the team is a great resource for any dietary questions, struggles, or concerns you might have, and they can usually meet with you right in the department. You can meet with them on an as-needed basis for the most part, but if you're struggling with eating food or significant weight loss, your oncologist might recommend that you meet with them more frequently for guidance and extra support.

<u>Researcher:</u> Depending on the department where you receive your care, participating in cancer research might be offered to you. You do not have to participate if you don't wish to—that, truly, is entirely up to you. But if you *are* interested, you can ask your radiation oncologist what your participation in the research would include. Sometimes it means a few meetings for a brief interview, sometimes it's blood work weekly or monthly, and sometimes it's simply filling out a questionnaire you can mail back.

Personal Story:

As I mentioned previously, I've had multiple family members with different cancer diagnoses. My father was diagnosed with prostate cancer a few years back. Luckily, his cancer was caught very early. He agreed to partic-ipate in a research study that included one meeting (about three hours long) to discuss, at length, his medical and life history as it would pertain to his diagnosis. I spoke with him after his meeting with the researcher, and he said, "You know, Margs, I was really surprised at the dedication to the minutiae that goes on behind the scenes. They explained to me what the goal of this research was and how they would use the information. They were telling me that this information would help them contribute to research and help move the collective forward as a cancer community. It was nice to gain a better understanding from an informed perspective, and it felt good to contribute to the research while getting relevant information about my own body relative to my care. You know, you don't know what's down the road, and it was nice to be able to get some information on where I could be going."

Participation in research isn't for everyone, but if you have an interest in your own body and body sciences and don't mind trading information with the researchers, you might surprise yourself with how good it can feel to get more information and to talk about it.

I have my consultation (first appointment) with the radiation oncologist. What should I expect?

Your radiation oncologist will present facts about your cancer and how it behaves. They will review any recent diagnostic medical imaging you might have had relative to your diagnosis to help establish exactly where the cancer is located in your body. They will review any surgical notes from your biopsy or other surgeries related to your diagnosis and make their best recommendations for treatment. This is your opportunity to make sure you communicate your goals for treatment and what is important to you.

As I've mentioned previously, there are multiple ways to create an effective, targeted, personalized, and comprehensive treatment plan for your cancer in *your* body specifically. This fact is not meant to discourage or overwhelm you by any stretch; rather, this idea should comfort you.

Radiation oncologists have a broad spectrum of knowledge to pull from and will be able to give you their best recommendations for treatment. Rest assured that it is their job and their desire to be your information database for the most trusted, updated, and accurate information specific to your goals for treatment and the type of cancer you have. Information provided by your radiation oncologist will very likely be infinitely more reliable, helpful, and accurate than endless hours of Internet research.

This appointment is your opportunity to bring up your concerns, your goals, your future, your fears—any and all types of discussion are on the table. You should leave this appointment feeling as if you have left nothing unsaid or unasked. Any question you would type into an Internet search bar should be exactly what you bring to this appointment to get precise and accurate information pertinent to you specifically. It can also be helpful to write your questions down ahead of time and bring them to your appointment. If you don't know where to begin with questions for your oncologist, here are some to get you started:

- Have you treated this type of cancer before?

- How many treatments do I need if I'm seeking a cure?

- What are common side effects for treatment in this area?

- What can I do to alleviate the symptoms of these side effects if they occur?

- Would you recommend any other therapies in conjunction with the radiation?

- What are the latest clinical trials for my disease, and are there any that might be appropriate for me?

These are just a few suggestions to get the conversation started if you feel as if you need a little prompting. These physicians are highly trained to help you make big decisions about your cancer treatment choices. When you leave this appointment, you should be feeling on track, confident, and hopeful that there is an excellent and pinpointed strategy for you to move forward.

***

Let's take a moment and pause our walk at the shoreline.

Let's rest.

This was a lot of new and detailed information, so let's take a moment to digest it.

Slowly take a breath in as you acknowledge how good it feels to find your footing. You now know the right people to turn to for help, and that starts to slow down your scattered thoughts.

Gaining this understanding of how to approach your consultation has you feeling more prepared than you were before.

As you exhale, you can feel the tension in your muscles slowly release, because you now know a little bit more about what to expect from this process, as you've uncovered another piece of the unknown.

Take all the time you need here, and just breathe.

As we stand here together in the quiet calm, with the cold water at our feet, my thoughts slowly begin to wander back to those broken glass pieces, and I wonder what has become of them now.

Undoubtedly, the pieces have drifted apart through no fault of their own. Scattered and uncertain and at the mercy of the sea, they have little choice but to forge forward, though they are unsure of what's next.

When you're feeling ready, let's keep going.

4

CT Simulation

Designing Your Treatment Plan, Tips for Success,
and the Notorious Radiation Tattoos

If you decide to pursue radiation therapy, you will then be set up with your first appointment to prepare your personalized treatment: your CT simulation. This appointment is also referred to as *CT sim, mapping,* or a *planning session.*

What is the goal and purpose of the CT simulation appointment?

We will utilize a CT scanner to develop a three-dimensional picture solely for the purpose of radiation treatment planning. What makes this scan unique for our planning purposes is that this image is acquired in the *exact position* you will be in for your radiation treatment. This three-dimensional picture will allow us to visualize the area we will be treating, along with the general anatomy directly surrounding it. We use this scan to design exactly where the radiation will be delivered, allowing us to conceive a fine-tuned and highly detailed radiation treatment plan that is completely geared to you.

How is this CT scan different from one I might have had recently?

If you have had prior CT scans outside of this CT sim appointment, they are most likely *diagnostic quality* scans (meaning they were used to help diagnose disease). Although both types are referred to as CT scans, I assure you that these two scans are used for very different purposes. Diagnostic quality CT scans do not pay any regard to the position you're in when you're scanned and only help your HCP see inside your body to identify the location of any cancer. The CT simulation for radiation treatment planning is not for diagnosing but to precisely pinpoint the exact position you will be in for your radiation treatment.

How can I prepare for this appointment? For example, is there anything specific I should wear or avoid?

If there are any specific directives or requests from your team prior to your planning scan (eating, drinking, filling your bladder, etc.), they will be made very clear to you before your appointment, likely at your consultation. The directives for CT sim prep can vary depending on the area receiving treatment and the protocols in place within the department. It's best to check with your HCP ahead of this appointment if you have any doubts or questions regarding directives. If you haven't received any specific instructions, you can proceed without restrictions.

In terms of what to wear to this appointment, each department has its own set of preferences. Some facilities prefer that their patients change into hospital gowns regardless of the intended area for treatment, and other facilities might just have you remove a piece of clothing or metal that could interfere with the scan. Your team will direct you upon arrival.

In general, a good rule of thumb for this type of scan is to minimize any removable metal you could wear into the room. This would include belts, watches, jewelry, pins, and such—not because of any looming dangers of physical interaction with the machine but for the utmost scan quality, personal item security, and appointment efficiency.

We will ask you to remove any metal in the area we will be scanning because this can create what we call an *artifact* on our image. This artifact can distort the clarity of our image, a less than desirable situation. If we can avoid it simply by removing metal before the scan, we will. Sometimes there are metal clips or stents placed within your body from surgery that obviously can't be removed for the scan. Please don't worry; in these instances, we have a work-around in our treatment planning system to address these image quality circumstances.

For security purposes, it's usually best to leave expensive personal items or jewelry at home if you don't feel comfortable removing them and storing them in a locker at the clinic. Arriving with fewer items to keep track of, to remove, or to fuss with can make things that much easier for you and allow you to focus on what is important at this appointment.

It seems simple, but I've seen nerves get the best of people as they try to remove these items in a hurry—they're worried about removing multiple items quickly, what's going to happen next, and where they're going to store the items. To simplify things for yourself, try not to wear multiple layers of clothing and, if possible, keep removable metal and jewelry to a minimum. Empty your pockets ahead of time.

Although these specific CT sim prep tips aren't imperative for successful completion of your planning session, they can certainly contribute to streamlining your experience and decreasing your stress.

What can I expect to experience at the CT simulation?

You can expect to be instructed and assisted by the radiation therapist as to the exact position we will have you in for your CT sim and your subsequent treatments. Depending on what area of your body is receiving treatment, an *immobilization device* might be created for you, or you may receive *tattoos* at this appointment (more on these to follow). The radiation therapists will take great care in positioning you for this scan, so please be patient with them, as sometimes it can take some time to decide on optimal positioning.

Once your positioning has been established, you will notice your team documenting the specifics of *exactly how we have you positioned* for this scan. This documentation can include written information, such as specific measurements and settings for positioning devices included in your treatment setup. Additionally, pictures can be taken with a digital camera to document your exact positioning and any markings they've made on your skin or immobilization device. These pictures aid significantly in assuring your setup can be fine-tuned for reproducibility and consistency. As the saying goes, "Pictures are worth a thousand words," and in our line of work, these pictures provide support for nuances in positioning that help us ensure we can achieve our highly desired to-the-millimeter precision. Thorough documentation for this appointment is integral and is the responsibility of your treatment team. You will never be asked to reproduce your treatment position on your own, so don't worry about trying to remember the details.

The longest part of this CT sim appointment is selecting the particulars for your positioning as well as the precise nature of our documentation. It is very likely that the actual scan itself will be the quickest part of your appointment.

What is an immobilization device?

The goal of an immobilization device is to stabilize and isolate the area of the body we want to treat. Effective immobilization can help us avoid the areas we don't want to irradiate. Sometimes your CT scan might include very specific positioning that doesn't necessitate an immobilization device. It's important to know that we don't always make an immobilization device for every area of the body we can treat. Sometimes positioning alone can be successful in achieving our setup goals. Immobilization devices and radiation therapy positioning equipment can vary by facility and treatment type. When you go to your consultation, you can ask your physician how you will be positioned and if you should expect any custom immobilization devices.

What is happening behind the scenes at the
CT simulation appointment?

Your radiation oncologist is telling the radiation therapists exactly what area(s) of the body they want to treat, indicating what anatomy they want included in the CT scan (in order to gather information about the surrounding structures), and also addressing any concerns or specifics they might have regarding your positioning or challenges with mobility, and so on.

What are the clinician's goals for this appointment,
and how do they affect me as a patient?

The main objective of this appointment from the clinician's perspective is to find a balance between these two facets: helping patients get into a comfortable body position so they can *hold still* for the duration of their treatment while simultaneously taking care to ensure *utmost reproducibility* of your body position. You see, a highly reproducible treatment position sets both patients and the treatment team up for success moving forward. When patients are relatively comfortable in the treatment position, it is likely they will lie very still. With cooperation from patients in this manner, we can increase consistencies in our measurements from day to day, subsequently allowing us to provide more efficient treatment delivery as well. When we can deliver effective and precise treatment efficiently, patients generally have a more positive treatment experience. This is a highly desirable goal, both from the patient's and staff's perspective, and one we focus on as a team consistently.

Tattoos Explained

If there is one aspect about radiation therapy that people are generally aware of, it's that you might get tattooed. Without knowing any background about why this is the case, it's hard not to find yourself imagining the worst. *Not only do I have to get radiation, but now I'm going to be tattooed as well? Wait—permanently marked? Is that what they mean? How big are these tat-*

toos, and where are they going to be on my body? What do the tattoos look like, and why do I need them?

I understand that without any additional information, the word *tattoo* carries a certain stigma. Allow me to uncover all the details about radiation tattoos.

What do the tattoos look like, and what's the purpose of them?

The tattoos are permanent markings we make on our patients that consist of very tiny ink dots placed just under the surface layer of your skin. Often the size of a very small freckle, these tattoos help the radiation therapists get you into the correct position for treatment and assist in directing accurate measurements for your treatment setup.

The tattoo placement on your body is not necessarily indicative of *exactly where* the radiation is going; rather, they serve two important purposes. Aiding the radiation therapists in achieving our goals of the highly valued *position reproducibility*, the tattoos help us get you into the same position you were in for your CT sim. Next, the tattoos provide a pinpointed and distinct location that radiation therapists utilize in order to apply millimeter measurements provided by the radiation oncologist from the directives of your treatment plan.

If I don't get tattoos, how will the radiation therapists know how to position me for treatment or where to direct the radiation?

If you don't receive tattoos for treatment, that is very much okay. This could mean there are markings on your immobilization devices that we will use in place of any tattoos. Or this could mean the clinic where you're receiving your treatment has technology or processes in place that utilize other tools to establish the correct treatment position and don't require tattoos. Historically, radiation tattoos have been imperative in delivering accurate radiation treatments; however, treatment technology has now evolved and become so efficient that there are areas of the body we can treat accurately without needing tattoos. You can ask your radiation oncologist if you should expect to receive any tattoos for your treatment and what process they have in place to assure that your treatment is delivered accurately each day.

The tattoos are so tiny! How can the treatment team tell exactly which marks on my body are the tattoos?

You might wonder how we can see these marks, as they really are incredibly small. The tattoos have an inky blue tint to them, delineating them from any freckles you may have, which are usually brown in tone. Most important, we place these tattoos strategically on your body, so we know where to look for them.

Are these tattoos permanent, and can I have them removed?

Yes, the tattoo markings are permanent, but they do naturally fade over time. If you're bothered by the sight of these tattoos, after your treatment has been completed (and with approval from your radiation oncologist), you can get them removed—although this is not common and not recommended. There is a disadvantage to removing these tattoos, and I would be remiss if I didn't explain why.

If it is ever decided that you will receive radiation to an adjacent area in the future, the tattoos could be very valuable in assisting your treatment team in keeping you as safe as we possibly can. We will use the old tattoos to re-create the details of your previous radiation treatment plan on our special treatment planning software, which allows us to track where the radiation has already been delivered. This is important in assisting your team in developing a concrete understanding of how much radiation certain tissues and organs have already received. We have an obligation as your treatment team to keep you safe from the radiation, and the previous tattoos can assist us in doing just that.

Fun Fact: As radiation therapy students, it is not uncommon for us to practice our tattooing technique on ourselves. Years ago, I did just that and gave myself a tattoo on the side of my hand. In a discussion about radiation treatment with a girlfriend I've had since my elementary school years, I showed her the tattoo on the side of my hand. She told me she had genuinely never noticed it—further proving my point about how small the tattoos really are and how visually insignificant they can be to someone who isn't looking for them.

Alleviating Anticipatory Worries about the CT Simulation

Please don't let anticipatory feelings of body aches or pains worry or stop you from moving forward with your CT simulation. I can assure you that your treatment team has a lot of experience with people who have difficulties with lying flat, claustrophobia, body-image sensitivities, modesty, tight or stiff muscles from surgery, limited mobility, painful joints and bones, and so on. We run into these challenges constantly in our work, and we have all the tools to make sure we can get you comfortable and in a position that is highly reproducible for your treatment. If you're struggling with physical pain or mental anxieties, please speak up and mention this to your radiation oncologist or radiation nurse. We have multiple options to help you lie comfortably still for this scan, and we will be happy to come up with a helpful solution for you. Once you are relatively comfortable, it is highly likely that your position will be reproducible—and this should be your number one takeaway from this appointment.

Tips for Success at This Appointment

I want to make sure that I'm very clear here: please let your team know if anything is painful for you as you're working with them to establish your treatment position. Your positioning shouldn't be *painful* for you, but it might be a little *uncomfortable*. This discomfort can present itself physically, because sometimes the positioning can feel a little awkward or unnatural for you, and mentally, because taking the steps through this whole cancer treatment process can certainly feel overwhelming at times—understandably so. You can ask your radiation therapist how long you should expect to be in this position. The time can range anywhere from five to thirty minutes, depending on the type of treatment you're having. On average, treatment usually takes between ten and fifteen minutes to deliver, and CT simulation times can be anywhere from fifteen to forty-five minutes.

I hope this information allows you to successfully advocate for yourself if anything about this part of the process feels intolerable for you. We are here as a team to work *with you* in getting your cancer treated. It is ideal if you can relax your body and release muscular tension *before* the scan, as this can be helpful in reproducing your positioning. Without lifting your body off the table, wiggling, or moving your arms and legs, try taking a breath in through your nose and slowly exhaling through your mouth—this can release any extra tension you might not have realized you had. During the scan, it's important that you breathe normally, unless instructed otherwise. Please don't worry, though, if you're unable to relax or are carrying muscle tension or stress. I will explain how we manage slight discrepancies in your positioning to ensure we're treating exactly where we intend for every treatment. After all, we recognize that we're working with people, not square boxes. We have processes and procedures in place to help us ensure accurate treatment delivery even if your position is minutely different each time. You will learn more about this in chapter 5, "Receiving Radiation Treatment."

I've completed the CT simulation. What happens next?

At the end of your CT sim appointment, it is very likely that you'll receive a date to return to begin your treatment, and in some departments they might give you the entirety of your treatment schedule (dates and times) at this appointment. The next time you come back to the department will be for your first radiation treatment appointment, often referred to as a *virtual simulation* or *V-sim*. You will learn about the details of this appointment in chapter 5, "Receiving Radiation Treatment."

Once this CT sim appointment has been completed, that's when we really get to work behind the scenes designing your individualized radiation treatment plan. The design of this plan can take anywhere from a few days to two weeks, and this is the reason behind the delay in starting radiation treatment. Your start-date timeline can vary based on the urgency and intricacy of your treatment and will ultimately be determined by your radiation oncologist.

Resimulation: Why Might This Happen? What Is It For?

A resimulation is simply an appointment for another CT simulation, often referred to as a *rescan*. If this is required, please don't be alarmed. There are a few different reasons why your treatment team might ask you to participate in a resimulation.

Boost simulation: Sometimes, as part of your complete radiation course of treatment, your radiation oncologist will prescribe a *boost* or a *cone down*. This means that they're planning on shrinking the size of the treatment area, making it smaller and a little more focused. The boost treatment can sometimes be focused on the area from which a tumor was removed, called the *surgical bed*.

The new three-dimensional image acquired at this appointment can help your treatment team accurately determine this smaller area of focus. Also, sometimes we will reposition you for your boost treatment, and this scan allows us to gather a three-dimensional picture of you in this new position for treatment planning purposes.

Significant tumor-size changes: If there are significant changes in tumor size within the area of treatment, your radiation oncologist might request that you have a resimulation. This will create a new three-dimensional image to ensure the radiation dose coverage is appropriate and still effectively treating the intended area.

If there is significant tissue swelling, sometimes it can make some custom immobilizations uncomfortable, and a new immobilization can be created. In this instance, a new immobilization would prompt a new

CT image to be acquired, and thus, a resimulation.

Sometimes the tumor itself might be very responsive to treatment and could shrink significantly. This is great news, but it can sometimes result in an ill-fitting immobilization that could impact the dose delivery. This could also result in the need for a new immobilization to be created, which in turn would require a resimulation so a new three-dimensional picture can be attained.

Adjusting your treatment position if you find it intolerable to lie still: Sometimes, due to unforeseen circumstances, you might find that you're unable to lie still in the position you were in for your original CT simulation. If significant adjustments need to be made to your position and these changes impact the positioning of the area intended for treatment, it is likely that your team will bring you back into the planning room for another CT scan.

If the positioning adjustment made does not impact the area receiving treatment, sometimes very minor adjustments can be made without needing resimulation, but this is not recommended. Remember, the objective of a CT sim is to acquire a scan of you in *the exact position for treatment,* so if we make alterations to your positioning after your CT simulation (especially directly relating to the exact area we're treating), it is likely we'll need to acquire a new CT image to ensure accurate treatment.

Designing a Radiation Treatment Plan: Behind the Scenes

The radiation treatment plan (often referred to as your *plan*) gets created behind the scenes in the time between your CT sim and your first radiation appointment. Your presence is not needed while this design is happening, as the plan is created utilizing the three-dimensional image acquired at your CT simulation appointment. Your treatment team can spend anywhere from a few hours (in emergent cases) to up to two weeks developing, designing, and performing rigorous quality-assurance checks to produce a highly customized treatment plan for you.

Who develops and designs the radiation treatment plan?

The radiation oncologist is the one who enters the directive for this plan. They dictate the total radiation dose you will receive, how many treatments you will receive to achieve that total dose, and how much dose you will receive each day. Your radiation oncologist will also be responsible for deciding what anatomy gets included in the area to be irradiated. They will work very closely with a medical dosimetrist to create the perfect treatment plan for you.

The medical dosimetrist is responsible for creating and designing your personalized radiation treatment plan based on directives from your radiation oncologist. Their goal is to create a treatment plan that effectively delivers the prescribed radiation to very specific areas while simultaneously minimizing dosage to the surrounding healthy tissues.

What goes into designing a radiation treatment plan?

Using a computer software program specifically designed for radiation treatment planning, your radiation oncologist and medical dosimetrist will work together to create a custom treatment plan for you. Consideration will be given to any recent diagnostic imaging studies you might have had, as well as any recent surgeries. They evaluate exactly where the cancer is located and then will plan the field of radiation to include the tumor and a small—meaning millimeter(s)—margin of healthy tissue directly surrounding it.

The exact margin of healthy tissue surrounding your tumor is dictated by your radiation oncologist and the type of radiation treatment you're having. I understand that including a margin of healthy tissue can sound a little intimidating; however, this margin is imperative for including all the cancer cells *in the area we irradiate* so we can ensure effective radiation treatment.

Once the area identified for radiation treatment is established, the medical dosimetrist chooses the angles of the radiation beam. They take great care in deciding where the beam will enter and exit the body and how they can avoid certain structures while treating the planned area effectively. The medical dosimetrist is highly trained to ensure your safety while simultaneously considering treatment-delivery efficiencies when they're constructing your treatment plan.

I provide these background details to you not to overwhelm or concern you but to help you understand the multiple layers of delivering safe and effective treatment for you. Please know that many considerations are taken throughout each phase of the treatment planning process to ensure that strict safety standards are maintained.

What are the different types of external beam radiation techniques, and how do I know which one is right for me?

There are multiple different types of external beam radiation treatment techniques, and even as this book goes to print, there are new protocols and treatment types being developed that could potentially become the new standard of care. For the most up-to-date treatments offered, I suggest you look to the American Cancer Society for their information regarding this topic. They do a great job describing and differentiating the types of radiation treatment.

Remember, you should use this information to provide yourself with a little background so when you meet with your oncology treatment team, they can direct you to the most appropriate treatment for your circumstances. Try not to concretely decide on one treatment before you've spoken with your experts.

***

Let's take a moment and pause our walk at the shoreline.

We're starting to get into the information about the actual treatment process. It can be a lot to take in, so let's take a moment to rest.

Slowly take a deep breath as you recognize how good it feels to have the ability to prepare yourself. You feel a little more relieved knowing what to expect from your planning session and your meeting with the radiation oncologist. This knowledge gives you strength as well as a little more courage to take these first steps.

Exhale the fear that does not serve you.

Take the time you need here. Just breathe.

As we stand peacefully together on this beach, with the smell of salt in the air, thoughts of that broken bottle emerge. It has been some time now since its arrival on the ocean floor. These pieces have been taken in directions not of their choosing but at the mercy of the current and tossed about by the unpredictable waves—some small and gentle, and others not so much.

Take your time here, and when you feel ready, let's keep walking.

5

Receiving Radiation Treatment

The First Radiation Appointment, What to Expect Before and During Your Treatment, and Positional Imaging Demystified

The First Radiation Appointment

It is likely a week or two has passed since you were in the department for your CT sim, and now you're coming back for your first radiation appointment. Good for you for taking charge and taking actionable steps to put this all behind you. Let me walk you through what these first few appointments could look like for you.

What is the importance of the first radiation appointment, referred to as a *virtual simulation* or *V-sim*?

The V-sim appointment is designed as a dry run for your treatment, meaning we are checking to ensure that your position is reproducible and that we can execute your treatment appropriately. This V-sim appointment is designed to verify treatment position and is not a radiation treatment. Sometimes the first treatment can be given at this same appointment if that is how you are scheduled by your team; however, most of the time, you will return the next business day to receive your first radiation treatment. You can ask your team if this appointment is just to verify positioning or if you will also be receiving the actual treatment.

What is the name of the radiation treatment machine, and what does it look like?

The machine that delivers the radiation treatment is called a *linear accelerator*. This machine is designed as an open space that can rotate around you but not touch you as you lie on a surface known as a *treatment couch* or *table*. A linear accelerator does not have an enclosed tube or doughnut-like opening to travel through, like an MRI or CT scan (great news for my claustrophobic readers).

The best way to see what the machine looks like before being in the department is to search the Internet for *linear accelerator*. There are a few different vendors for linear accelerators, so the style and capabilities of each machine will vary, but the design is relatively the same. Additionally, radiation oncology departments will sometimes show pictures of their treatment machines on their department website. If you have decided on a facility, you can likely find specifics about their treatment machines directly from them on their website.

Who delivers the radiation treatments?

The radiation therapists are the people who will escort you into the treatment room, position you for treatment, ensure you're in the correct position, and deliver the radiation treatments.

How does the radiation therapist know exactly what area to irradiate each time?

The radiation therapist will utilize the information from your treatment plan and CT simulation to ensure appropriate treatment each time. The radiation dose, shape of the radiation field, and angles of the machine for treatment delivery have already been meticulously determined by your radiation treatment plan. These specifics are preprogrammed into your radiation treatment chart. It's the job of the radiation therapist to make sure your positioning, or *setup*, each day is such that the preprogrammed custom plan will align perfectly on your body, thus ensuring a properly executed radiation treatment.

Will my radiation oncologist be present for my radiation treatment?

The radiation oncologist will not typically be present at the time of your treatment, as their role is more in the design and direction of the treatment, not the daily delivery.

Exceptions to this include certain types of high-dose radiation treatment where they would be present for treatment delivery but not necessarily in the room for treatment setup. Additionally, sometimes the radiation therapist will request that the physician stop by the treatment machine briefly if there's a quick question regarding your positioning or a certain skin reaction you might be experiencing, for example.

Before Radiation Treatment Is Delivered

What should I expect for my first time in the radiation treatment room?

You'll be escorted into the treatment room by a radiation therapist who will likely first verify that the information we have pulled up for you is correct. We can do this verbally by asking you your name, birthday, or address. Sometimes you will receive a card with a barcode and your name on it, which you'll scan to open up your chart. This first step is dependent on each department and their policies, but feel free to ask your team how they're ensuring that *your* chart is open.

I've found that people can grow tired of us asking these questions every day (and sometimes they get a bit irritated by the repetition), but really, this is an important initial step for each treatment and part of our process.

Once we verify this information, we'll get you into the same exact position you were in when you had your CT sim. Remember, you don't need to worry about recalling exactly how you were positioned—that's your team's responsibility.

How do the radiation therapists get me into the right position for treatment when we are inside the room?

The radiation therapists will assist you over to the treatment table and help guide you into the same position based on the documented information from your planning session. You will recognize the positioning devices or immobilizations from your CT sim. Depending on the area designated for treatment, the technology at your department, and the immobilization devices used, your radiation therapist will fine-tune your positioning until they are satisfied with the reproducibility. Please be patient with us when we are in the room making these adjustments. We are quite particular in order to provide you with the most effective treatment, and we work in millimeters, so you can imagine that sometimes this can take us a little time. Once your team is satisfied with your positioning, they will inform you of this and exit the treatment room.

During Radiation Treatment

Where do the radiation therapists go when they leave the treatment room?

Once your position has been reproduced in the treatment room, the team will head to an area directly adjacent to the room you are in called a *treatment console area*. We have cameras here so we can see you and the treatment machine the entire time, and we have a two-way audio box so we can freely communicate with you as well. These are requirements set by commissioning agencies that are nonnegotiable tools in a radiation therapy treatment room and treatment console area. Feel free to ask your radiation therapists to show you where they sit when delivering the treatments, if knowing makes you feel more comfortable. Often, you will walk right by the treatment console area when heading into the treatment room.

Although you will be in the room by yourself for a short period of time, there are still means to communicate with your treatment team if your need feels immediate. Since we don't want you to move once your team exits the treatment room, you can ask your team what their preference is for you to get their attention (if you require immediate assistance) when they're not in the room with you. Don't be shy about asking if you'd feel more comfortable having a clearly communicated plan in place.

The therapists have me in the correct position in the treatment room, and they have left to go to the treatment console area. Now what should I expect?

Depending on the type of treatment you are having, the next steps will vary. Sometimes we can go right into treatment delivery, and other times we will take some X-rays to help further fine-tune your position before treatment begins. The protocol specific to you will vary on a case-by-case basis. Please ask your radiation therapists to explain to you what their process is for making sure they have you lined up correctly for treatment.

Positional Imaging Demystified

We can use positional imaging to further improve upon your treatment setup before treatment begins specific to that day. Sometimes it is used before each treatment to fine-tune where the treatment will be delivered, and sometimes it's not used before each treatment. Your treatment team will be able to best explain the specifics regarding your personalized treatment delivery process, so you can ask them what you should expect for your treatment each time.

The equipment we use for positional imaging is attached to the linear accelerator. If you are receiving positional imaging, you'll be holding the same position through treatment setup, positional imaging, and treatment delivery, in that order.

What are some different types of positional imaging for radiation therapy treatment?

There are a few different types of imaging we can use before the treatment is delivered to further fine-tune treatment positioning. The appropriateness of imaging protocols will be different depending on treatment types and areas of the body. You can ask your radiation therapist what type of imaging they are using to verify your position and how often you can expect this imaging to occur.

CBCT (Cone Beam CT): This is a low-dose CT image that has been equipped specifically to cooperate directly with the linear accelerator. This image provides us with a three-dimensional picture of the exact position you are *currently in*, allowing us to make millimeter adjustments to that position to ensure adequate dose coverage for the intended area of that day's treatment.

Portal Films: This type of imaging produces a two-dimensional picture that is like that of a routine X-ray. We can also fine-tune your position with millimeter adjustments before treatment with this type of imaging.

SGRT (Surface-Guided Radiation Therapy): This is a technology that does not use radiation for image production—rather, it uses technology that reads the surface of your skin to align your body for treatment. We can use this for initial positioning as well as monitoring throughout radiation treatment delivery.

If I am being "imaged" every day as part of my radiation treatment, what can I expect?

Once the team has you set up in the treatment room, we will then proceed to the console area and take an image. When we take these images, *we are not looking to diagnose any disease*. The only goal of this daily imaging is to fine-tune your *treatment position* by identifying the millimeter adjustments we want to make *for that day's treatment* specifically. Once those adjustments have been selected, we will move the couch you are lying on to get you into the perfect position for treatment. You'll hold the same position for your setup in the treatment room, acquiring and analyzing the image, and for treatment delivery. Your team will employ the adjustment capabilities of the treatment couch to tweak your position for treatment delivery.

Depending on the equipment in the department, the radiation therapist might come into the treatment room and move the treatment couch themselves, or they might have this capability from outside the treatment room. Either way, you might notice the table you're lying on sounds or feels as if it's moving a little bit—you just keep holding still, as things are moving along great and your treatment delivery is going just as planned.

If my treatment type doesn't require daily imaging, what can I expect?

If you're not having daily imaging for positioning, the radiation therapists have other ways to ensure your position is precise before treatment delivery. You can ask them to explain what they check to ensure the appropriate position for treatment, as this can vary depending on the area designated for treatment. If your imaging protocol is not daily, they'll be taking positioning imaging weekly (technically, every five to seven treatments) to confirm all the different information they check daily is reliable and appropriate.

It wasn't planned for me to have positional imaging done today, but the radiation therapists took images anyway. What does this mean?

Although there are standard imaging protocols in place for your treatment, you might find that sometimes you will be imaged outside of your routine imaging schedule. Don't worry if this happens. In fact, you should feel encouraged by this. This means the radiation therapists might not be satisfied with your position in the treatment room, and they want to take an image to confirm the appropriateness of your setup before treatment begins. From this image, we can either verify everything is lined up perfectly and begin treatment, or we can adjust as necessary. As a professional cohort, radiation therapists are highly trained to not hesitate in making decisions that will support precise treatment delivery each and every time.

They've positioned me in the room and have taken the positioning X-rays. Now I'm lying here, and it feels like nothing is happening. What is going on?

Immediately after the X-rays have been taken, the radiation therapists will analyze the image just taken to ensure appropriate alignment for treatment that day. Analyzing this image is arguably the most important part of your treatment process, and this can take some time.

The amount of time to analyze this image can vary depending on the type of image taken and the area of the body designated for treatment. Expect that the amount of time to analyze the image will be different each day, as your positioning will be minutely different every time. Some days you might lie down and everything lines up very smoothly, and other days it will take us a few minutes to analyze and adjust your position to get it just right.

Roughly, it can take anywhere from ten seconds to four or five minutes to analyze this image and confidently identify the adjustments we want to make to your positioning. Once the therapists define the adjustments they desire to make to your position, they'll be able to move the table you are lying on and continue to treatment.

Ready for Treatment Beam

I'm in the perfect position and ready for treatment. What can I expect when the treatment radiation is being delivered?

Making sure we have you in the correct position and verifying all our information before we deliver the treatment is the longest part of your appointment. Delivering the actual treatment beam of radiation is the quickest. You won't feel anything when the radiation beam is on. You might hear the machine making some buzzing noises, much like the noises of a diagnostic X-ray machine. The machine will likely rotate around you, but it won't touch you. It's important to keep lying still until you hear one of the team members tell you the treatment has been completed. Feel free to ask your treatment team how long they expect your treatment to take, as each treatment is very different and customized for you, as you well know by now.

Helpful Tip to Support Peace of Mind for Daily Treatment

Remember, we're working with aligning treatment for *people*, not plastic boxes whose shape never changes. Our weight, our mobility, our range of motion, our skin elasticity, our muscle tension, our bloating, and our breathing patterns can fluctuate every day. These factors can influence your medical team's choices for your treatment process each day.

We *expect* there to be very minor differences in how you lie down on the table and how we position the exterior of your body in the treatment room each day. You will likely experience some days when you feel like your body is not quite in the *exact* same position, and this is okay.

Remember, we set very particular millimeter margins based on your treatment type within your treatment plan around the known area where cancer cells are present. These margins support your oncology team in ensuring we accommodate for these minute positioning discrepancies and that we are encompassing the targeted cancer cells within our treatment field for every treatment, regardless of daily positional imaging.

Your radiation therapists are highly trained to assess the circumstances and appropriateness for treatment each time, and it's their responsibility to make judgment calls for decisions that continually substantiate precise radiation treatment *each* time.

Treatment Scheduling

Do I need to be treated at the same time every day?

If your radiation oncologist has prescribed only one treatment a day for you, then the general answer to this question is no, you don't need to be treated at the same time every day. The exception to this rule is if your physician has prescribed two treatments a day for you. In that scenario, your treatment times will likely be dictated by your team to ensure the appropriate number of hours between treatments is achieved for maximum effectiveness of the radiation.

As a general rule of thumb, it's likely you'll be scheduled at or around the same time for your treatment each day. If you have a conflict that arises with your treatment time for a particular day, just let your radiation therapists know and they'll work to accommodate you for that change as best they can. Additionally, if your schedule is flexible and you're willing to accommodate potential time change requests from other patients, you can inform your team of your flexibility as well. Please let me be very clear that this is by no means necessary, required, or expected of any of our patients.

Treatment Scheduling Challenges Your Team Faces and Why This Can Affect Our Patients

As an oncology department, we have a responsibility to all our patients to provide equitable treatment time offerings for everyone; however, there are many intricacies to treatment scheduling that can influence availabilities for treatment times. These include departmental hours of operation, allocating designated time in our schedule for specialized treatment procedures, staff meetings, accommodating patients' alternative time requests, and collaborative meetings for physicians. I would be remiss if I didn't mention the unforeseen circumstances that cause treatment delays as well. These can include accommodating late patient arrivals, providing extra TLC for emotionally overwhelmed or sick patients, challenging treatment setups that require unexpected additional time to make sure we get them right, mechanical delays for repairs of our treatment equipment, and so on. Rarely are two days ever the same for the staff in a radiation oncology department.

I'm sharing this with you because it's important for you to understand that delivering safe and effective treatment is our number one priority every single day, minute to minute, unwaveringly. In order to accomplish this clinical goal and keep our high standards for quality treatment, sometimes the team can run behind schedule. While we are highly skilled in managing the intricacies of our treatment schedule and do our best to identify scheduling challenges ahead of time, sometimes unforeseen occurrences can cause delays that admittedly do affect our patients.

***

Let's take a moment and pause our walk at the shoreline.

Let's sit with this information—and rest.

Inhale the fresh air deeply, acknowledging how good it feels to have answers about this process and how proud of yourself you feel for facing this head-on.

Exhale fear and anxiety, as you now have facts and no longer fear this unknown.

Take a moment to acknowledge that you have chosen to no longer let fear lead. You are growing smarter and stronger through knowledge. You can sense a well-deserved calming energy, knowing you have created this new well of strength for yourself.

I smell the brininess of the ocean in our moment of peaceful pause, and I find my mind pondering those scattered glass pieces again. Time and the ocean's currents have pushed them to drift apart as they maneuver across the ripples of sand on the ocean floor. With encounters from the grit of each grain of sand, the glass begins to slowly exchange some of its sharp edges for softer ones.

Take all the time you need here.

When you're feeling ready, let's keep walking.

6

Managing Anxiety in the Treatment Room

How to Get through the Next Fifteen Minutes

Even with all the explanations and reassurance, sometimes people just really aren't comfortable at all with this process. That I can understand. Truthfully, the best way you can help your radiation therapists get you through the treatment as seamlessly and as quickly as possible is to lie as still as you can and try to relax. I'm sure you're thinking, *Is she serious?! That is easier said than done.* I promise, I hear you.

When people become anxious in the treatment room, I've found it's usually brought on by an overpowering tidal wave of uncertainties within the person—uncertainty about what to expect in the treatment room, uncertainty about the side effects, and uncertainty about their future. These uncertainties are real, and to say they can be overwhelming is an understatement. I've seen the look wash over people's faces—they're trying to listen to instructions or questions, but their mind is racing and going elsewhere. Trying to navigate a cancer diagnosis is a deeply personal experience, one that everyone has license to handle differently. Remember, your feelings surrounding these treatments are valid. That rush of emotion, the speed of your thoughts, and the reality of your circumstances can sometimes feel insurmountable in the moment. If this sounds like you, trust me when I say you are not alone.

When anxiety erupts like this, it can be challenging to find a way to quiet your *mind* so your *body* can relax. One method I've seen help people push past this anxiety in the treatment room is a shift in focus. Instead of trying to get answers for all the questions in your head, focus on one thing: getting through treatment *today*.

In this moment, you don't need to make a decision about receiving the next treatment—or even completing the treatments altogether. Your goal is to get through *just* this one, right now, today. Set your mind and make it your goal to successfully get this *one* treatment completed.

When you're feeling overwhelmed by the magnitude of this whole process, it can be very helpful to break it down into smaller accomplishments. Setting these smaller, achievable goals is powerful in mentally building your confidence and creating momentum. By successfully completing this one appointment, you've proven to yourself that you can do this. This fact will snowball your confidence into believing you can get through the next treatment and the one after that too. I have seen first-hand how effective this mindset can be in helping incredibly fearful and anxious patients get through their treatments.

Receiving cancer treatment can be a wildly emotional process. If a few tears spring up in the treatment room, know that you're not the first person and you certainly won't be the last. But I can tell you this: most people I've met in this capacity are *much* stronger than they give themselves credit for. I'm serious! You might surprise yourself with how much you can push past and continue to move forward. I've seen a number of patients have a significantly easier time once they have the first few treatments under their belt, as they now have a better idea of what to expect. A *piece* of the unknown is a little more known, right? Take comfort in that knowledge.

The Rule of 51 Percent

I came across this method from keynote speaker and author Jen Gottlieb in her book *BE SEEN*. While discussing the topic of how to conquer fear and move forward with confidence, she refers to "The Rule of 51 Percent." I couldn't help but draw parallels and inspiration from this for managing anxiety in the treatment room.

Gottlieb explains that we don't need to have 100 percent confidence in order to move forward or make a decision. If that were the case, we would seldom take action! She explains that the key to this rule of 51 percent is to "believe in ourselves a little bit more than we don't. Fifty-One Percent." Believing just *that* much more in ourselves will tip the scales and allow us to take action. How powerful! She also recognizes that this confidence percentage will fluctuate:

> *If you can convince yourself to take a tiny action, just the littlest baby step toward your goal, you're going to collect that win, celebrate, and add some dough to your confidence bank. Suddenly, you're at 52 percent and ready to act again. Before you know it, you're at 60 percent . . . 65 percent . . . 75 percent. One day, you might find you're up to 97 percent, and the next day you might drop back to 80. But the rule of 51 percent is all about knowing that's okay. It's about knowing where you are and giving yourself the grace to move forward, use your knowledge of that spectrum to keep your momentum going, and take action today . . .*[11]

Personally, I love this theory, because I feel like it grows confidence from a place of authenticity and allows us to move forward, even when we might not be feeling fully confident. Just believe in yourself one percent more than you don't—so simple yet so incredibly powerful for pushing through fear, gaining momentum, and building confidence.

Task Your Mind by Focusing Your Thoughts

It is no secret that the conversation you have with yourself in your head affects your reality—that is true even outside of a cancer diagnosis. Since my goal here is to help you get through your radiation treatments, I can

---

[1] Jen Gottlieb, BE SEEN: *Find Your Voice, Build Your Brand, Live Your Dream* (Carlsbad, California: Hay House Inc., 2023), 52–53.

offer you some advice for your headspace while you're on the table actively receiving your radiation treatment.

Some people find it helpful to check out mentally while in the room. To do this, think about any place that brings you joy. Imagine it vividly with smells, sights, and sounds, then envision yourself there and mentally leave the treatment room.

It can also be helpful to think about how good it feels to be proactive in receiving treatment. You're strong and courageous enough to tackle your health challenges head-on, so give yourself some credit. Think about how proud you are for pushing past your fears and getting treatment. You're in the treatment room, and *you* are making this happen—believe it!

I've also known patients who choose this moment to meditate, focusing their thoughts on their strengths rather than their weaknesses— valuing their courage in seeking out and going through with treatment, loving themselves enough to do hard things, appreciating themselves for having the grit it takes to get through this and show up consistently, and acknowledging how strong their will is and how their body will follow suit to heal.

Don't underestimate the narrative you tell yourself for these fifteen minutes. This time has power. What thoughts are you giving power to? What do you want your narrative to sound like?

Covering or Closing Your Eyes

It might feel like a seemingly small suggestion, but I've seen how closing or covering one's eyes can help a person get past the physical anxieties surrounding machinery close by or feelings of claustrophobia. I can understand why the thought of a large machine rotating around you could make you nervous. If that's the case, sometimes it can be as simple as closing or covering your eyes. You can ask your team for a pillowcase or washcloth (we always have these handy in the treatment room), or you can bring in your own eye mask to wear.

Of particular note if you're being treated in the head or neck area: you might have to opt for closing your eyes instead of covering them, as the physical placement of an eye mask, washcloth, or pillowcase could interfere with your treatment beam or immobilization device. You can check with your team to see what your best options might be.

Audible Distractions

If you have a tough time focusing your thoughts, another great option is to distract yourself by focusing on listening instead.

Listening to music that you love and inspires you can be a very powerful diversion while you're receiving your radiation treatment. There's usually music playing in the radiation treatment room, either from a streaming service or the radio, so you can ask your treatment team if the music can be changed to your preference. It's a quick and easy fix to make you comfortable, and we're happy to do it. Alternatively, you can create your own playlist and play it on your phone, which can be placed at the end of the treatment table or on a chair nearby. I will caution you, though, that headphones really aren't ideal because we need to make sure you can hear us over the intercom if we want to communicate with you. It's also worth knowing that the walls in the treatment room are built to shield radiation, so good wireless Internet reception in the treatment room is not typical. If you're bringing your own music, make sure it's downloaded.

Another great option for distraction is listening to audiobooks. Immerse yourself in a great story, and let your mind go elsewhere for a few minutes. I've seen patients have terrific success with this technique.

Additionally, you can play some calming, wordless music if that helps you relax. We've turned the treatment room into a spa many times with that energy! This can sometimes help people focus on meditating and envisioning themselves successfully completing their treatment, showing gratitude to themselves that they are strong enough to face their health challenges head-on.

Comforts in a Modesty Drape

Sometimes this process leaves our modest patients feeling very uneasy and overexposed in the treatment room, making it very challenging for them to relax and lie still. Feeling overexposed in front of complete strangers and having to receive your cancer treatment at the same time can be incredibly uncomfortable. I'll let you know that we do need to uncover the area of your body we're delivering radiation treatment to in order to position your body properly; however, if an area of your body is not receiving treatment, we can usually provide you with a pillowcase, sheet, or larger blanket to cover up. It seems like a small thing, but it can really make a big difference in the level of comfort for some people. If you're feeling uncomfortably overexposed in the treatment room, ask your team what they can offer you to cover up a little bit more.

The Comfort of Warm Blankets

Blanket warmers are a common amenity that most radiation oncology centers utilize. Typically, readily accessible warm blankets are offered to patients receiving radiation treatments. Don't underestimate the power of a warm blanket in a cold hospital to make the few minutes of receiving your treatment that much more bearable. Warm blankets can be incredibly comforting and work well to take the edge off and help you relax.

If You Overheat When You Are Nervous

Some people run hot when they get nervous. Just the thought of lying perfectly still as sweat drips off can make you nervous all over again. You might be surprised by the power of a cold washcloth on your forehead, the back of your neck, your wrists, or your feet. It can do wonders to break that nervous cycle and allow your nerves to subside enough to relax your muscles and get through the next few minutes.

Also, some treatment facilities have a fan in the room that can create some air circulation and a much-needed breeze. If they don't have a fan in the room, a small, personal battery-operated fan at your feet on the end of the table would more than likely be agreeable with your team. It seems so simple, but this is often enough to relieve that edge of discomfort so you can relax enough to get through those few minutes during treatment.

The Power of a Sentimental Item

Some people bring in a small blanket, pillow, or stuffed animal that gives them peace and reminds them of their loved ones. Having a physical item that represents what motivates you to get through these treatments can be very powerful for conquering fears and pushing through to complete your treatments.

Conclusion

The biggest takeaway here is that there are multiple ways for us to help you get as comfortable as we possibly can. You might come up with something that's helpful to you and isn't listed above, so feel free to think outside the box. It can't hurt to ask your team to make a small adjustment for you, and if it doesn't interfere with the radiation beam or treatment delivery, I'm certain they would be happy to comply with your request. Remember, break down your thoughts and focus on one thing only: getting through *today's* treatment. That's it. Believe in yourself a little more than you don't. Don't let the magnitude of fear or the "cancer whirlwind" paralyze you into inaction. You can absolutely do this. One treatment, one day at a time.

***

Let's take a moment and pause our walk at the shoreline.

Acknowledge that this topic can be heavy, but our conversation doesn't have to be.

As you inhale, recognize how good it feels to *know* you have tools to help you manage your anxiety. You're preparing yourself, setting your intentions and expectations in your mind. It feels powerful to set yourself up for success.

Exhale as you release the tension of self-doubt. Feel how much lighter you can be without it.

Take the time you need here and just breathe. Slowly breathe in through your nose and then breathe out through your mouth even more slowly. As you do this, reflect on the tools that inspire strength in you to accomplish your goal.

As we stand at the ocean's edge together, with the strong smell of ocean brine and salt in the air, I think about those glass pieces and what has become of them now. Interactions with the sand and strong currents have softened those edges even further. With that softening comes the cold sting of salt water, that unrelenting brine that causes the glass to be stripped of its glossy finish and makes the glass dull, softer, and pitted over time. Without much choice but to continue as they are, the pieces brave the elements of the ocean.

I know you grow tired from the magnitude of new information. Keep going. You're so much stronger than you think.

Take as much time as you need, and when you feel ready, let's walk.

7

How to Support a Healthy Headspace

Nurturing Your Spirit and the Power of Perspective

Cancer diagnosis or not, what you tell yourself and the thoughts that go through your head are so powerful in contributing to your overall well-being. Sometimes the magnitude of the swirling thoughts in your head can be stronger than actual facts—this is a challenge we all face in just about every aspect of our lives.

Most people who know me would consider me an upbeat and optimistic person. I do believe this comes somewhat naturally for me, but it doesn't always. I, too, have had to work on my own headspace. Now I try to be a little more mindful about what I communicate to myself as *truth*. This concept is incredibly important, especially when undergoing radiation treatments. When you're up against a cancer diagnosis, it's natural for you to immediately think of the worst-case scenario, but it doesn't mean you can't reprogram your thoughts to better support your healing.

The Power of Your Own Experience

There are few things more powerful than the palpable truth of your own experience. I often witness a significant shift in people's energy and attitude once they know what to expect after having a few radiation treatments under their belt. Not knowing what to expect in any scenario can bring forth nerves and anxieties that otherwise might not be present; receiving radiation treatment is no different. The hard truth is you can often overcome these stressful feelings by facing them. Your own experience in getting through that first treatment will help you build trust in yourself that you can get through this. This trust you've created for yourself, in turn, builds confidence.

You're allowed the authenticity of your own experience. One bad moment or appointment can certainly trip you up, but don't let that dictate the rest of your experience. Brush yourself off, give yourself some grace, and believe that the next day can be different.

Feel Your Feelings

Trying to present yourself determinedly to the world (or your loved ones) as a pillar of strength can be really difficult if you don't really feel that way—yet. Trying to stay strong for yourself and your people is admirable. But, to be honest, if you're just burying your fears and emotions and not dealing with them, chances are they'll catch up to you. Holding on so tightly to this emotional burden can feel crushing, which is not ideal when you're striving to embody strength.

The emotional magnitude of a cancer diagnosis is a lot, to say the absolute least. I need you to know that it's okay to *feel* these feelings. In order to be strong, you have to be real, especially with yourself. You have to feel the feelings that come up for you: disappointment, anxiousness, frustration, fear, nervousness, anger, overwhelm, and so on. Whatever those emotions are for you, I need you to know that they're valid. I'll repeat that to you a few times in this book because it's so important to know. It's okay to acknowledge these feelings, and it's imperative you let them out. Talk to someone about them or write in a journal. The only way to not let your feelings run the show is to get them out of your system, your body, and your mind. If you don't, it's likely they'll push to the surface at the most inopportune and inconvenient times. Once you release your feelings, you'll find the control they hold over you has lessened significantly.

I know from experience that holding on to your feelings out of fear of burdening others, what might happen if you say them out loud, or experiencing shame for feeling a certain way will hurt you far more than it will help you. If the thought of releasing these emotions makes you uncomfortable, sometimes it can be helpful to set a time frame to let out those emotions you've been holding on to and actually lean into them. Maybe it's for the next hour or two or maybe even the rest of the day. Once you've acknowledged and released these feelings, they don't hold the power over you they once did. You're not weak for feeling. You're strong for facing and dealing with what's coming up for you, and I know after you do, you'll feel stronger for it. Once you acknowledge these feelings, they'll still be there on the sidelines, but they'll have far less power. Don't let your unexpressed emotions keep a powerful grip on your spirit.

Why It's Important to Drown Out the Noise

Upon a new cancer diagnosis, it can feel like everyone is quick to offer you advice based on someone else's experience with a certain treatment, doctor, hospital, and so on. I can't emphasize enough how important it is to remember that everyone's cancer circumstances are different and so are the intricacies of their treatment. Without being an oncology professional, it's difficult to understand the nuances surrounding choosing the correct treatment, physician, and so on. While friends and family might be quick to share stories of hardship or success because they know someone else with "the same cancer," I would urge you to take their stories with a grain of salt. Setting your expectations around someone else's experience can subconsciously be setting yourself up to anticipate someone else's challenges too. While our loved ones' intentions are pure, sometimes the abundance of opinions can muddy your thoughts. Be mindful of the source of your advice, and make sure you're somewhat cautious about what information you take to heart. Drown out the noise and opinions and listen to your oncology experts.

Lean on Your Experts

Once you start radiation treatment, it's inevitable that you will have questions as you move forward. I want to encourage you to lean on your care team for answers. Getting reliable answers to your questions is especially important as it relates to your health during treatment. We're experts in getting people through this, and we do so by providing our patients with information and answers to their questions so solutions or peace of mind can be obtained. The sooner you bring your concern to your treatment team, the quicker we can address it and get you feeling better.

You're not alone in your feelings or experiences because you have your team of experts ready and willing to help you. If you have a question about your radiation treatment or any side effect you might be feeling, asking your radiation therapist is a great place to start. You'll see them every day for your treatment, and they're a great, quick resource for you on a day-to-day basis. If they can't answer your question, they'll know exactly where to direct you so your concerns can be addressed.

The Power of Reframing Your Thoughts

I'm not here to lead you with blind positivity—that's cheap, especially when discussing cancer treatment. I'm here to tell you facts that will help evoke courage and confidence within yourself to complete your radiation treatment. As much as this can be hard to hear, you participate in your own experience, and while we can't control our bodies physically, we can influence our own headspace. Let's learn how to influence it to support healing.

At the clinic, my strongest efforts consistently surround nurturing the mental health of the patients in my care. I've found there is no greater power for a healthy headspace than having the *right* information at the right time. Using knowledge is wildly powerful in transforming a negative headspace. The power of appropriate information to support your experience can allow your brain to reframe your thinking from negative and overwhelmed to thoughts of clarity, understanding, and peace. This shift is brought about by the ability to see things in a different light.

Reframing Radiation—from Toxic Property to Healing Aid

I bet you're thinking, *How is she going to pull this one off? How am I supposed to reframe something from dangerous, toxic, and cancer-causing to healing?*

It's easy on the surface to look at radiation as something you'd want to stay away from. After all, we've always been taught that radiation is dangerous, and in combination with the scary bright radiation signs on the doors to the treatment room, it's no wonder this topic doesn't really give you warm and fuzzy feelings. Not to confuse you, but you're right. Radiation can be dangerous when mishandled and harmful when overexposure occurs; however, when we use radiation intentionally and therapeutically, it has proved to be an incredibly effective cancer treatment. Get ready for this knowledge to change how you feel about radiation treatments!

I'm going to take a few steps back here and start with the science of the *cell cycle process*. (I promise, this will be brief, and it's important to understand.) Your body's natural cell cycle process is a series of events that take place in a cell so it can grow and divide, producing more of the same cell. This natural process takes about two weeks to complete from beginning to end. When an external beam of therapeutic radiation encounters your body tissues, the radiation will damage the DNA of all the cells in its path—healthy cells and cancer cells. It sounds a little intimidating, I know. Stay with me.

Your body will go through its natural cell cycle process to repair the damaged cells successfully, but this repair process only works for the healthy cells, *not* the cancer cells. You see, cancer cells do not have the ability to repair themselves through the natural cell cycle process, therefore the radiation inhibits their ability to reproduce and effectively destroys their function. The radiation will stop the replication of new cancer cells within that field of radiation, and your body will naturally support regeneration of healthy new cells.

This scientific fact is one of the main reasons people report feeling tired with radiation treatment.

So, now that you have this background information, reframe your thoughts about the radiation. Radiation is not something that's fighting your body but rather a tool that's working *with* your body in support of healing itself—incredible! Let this new perspective powerfully shift your thinking from intimidated and afraid to informed and aware.

Fatigue and Its Effect on Your Spirit

You'll find I mention fatigue a few different times throughout this book. It's important to understand why you feel so tired when you're going through radiation treatments, as it's the number one side effect people experience. You've learned about the science of what causes physical fatigue; however, under this umbrella of headspace, I want to speak about the effects fatigue can have on your spirit.

Facing each day while trying to squeeze in a quick visit to the oncology department for your radiation treatment can grow monotonous and tiring. Knowing that this is one more thing to add to your already busy day can feel exhausting. I will not downplay that showing up five days a week for radiation can certainly contribute to overall fatigue. The mental orchestration to make that happen can be an added stressor in an already hectic time.

The second or third week of radiation is usually when the fatigue can start to catch up to our patients (although it's important to know that many factors affect this timeline). Your body is now well into its own healing through the cell cycle process. Although this process is completed subconsciously, it can still be draining. At this point in treatment, your skin can start to become bothersome (more on this later), and showing up for treatment can really start to feel like a chore. The combination of these things can easily have you feeling down.

At this stage, when mental and physical fatigue is really setting in, I find that people sometimes communicate this type of fatigue to their brain in the form of thoughts such as, *I don't know if I can do this. The cancer is going to win. I can't take much more of this. I should just throw in the towel now.* Feeling tired throughout radiation treatments has *nothing* to do with your mental fortitude or the strength of your own physical body.

Don't let fatigue make you feel like the cancer is winning—because it isn't! If that thought passes through your head, let it be fleeting, because you know the *scientific truth.* Your body is working overtime to repair itself from the repetitive treatments, and that subconscious process can pull a lot of energy from you. Remember, at this point, you're well into treatment and your body has been continuously working hard to do what it's trained to do. If you can honor your body by giving it the physical rest it needs and feed your mind with truth from science, you'll hold a powerful and peaceful space within yourself for healing.

The Power of an Experienced Ally and Mentor

There can sometimes be no greater validation than speaking with someone who has successfully made it through what you're going through right now. There's great power behind experience, and there's no better time to utilize this concept than when going through radiation treatments.

As much guidance, knowledge, and support as I can give you on the topic of receiving radiation treatments, I can't speak to you from a patient's point of view. Sometimes, no matter how much someone says they understand, there's nothing more powerful than speaking with a peer who can validate your emotions and experience. Also, it can be very encouraging to see someone in a similar situation complete their treatment and move on with their life.

I'll never forget the first time I witnessed how powerful authentic mentorship can be. For a few years of my career, I delivered a specialized external beam radiation treatment called *proton radiation therapy*. This type of radiation is great for people with intricately located tumors and pediatric patients due to the special properties of the radiation beam. Early on in my time working with this type of treatment, I witnessed a pediatric patient around the age of seven, who was undergoing radiation treatment to his brain, coach another child of his age who was scared and had yet to begin the treatment process. This brave kiddo under treatment confidently walked his new friend into the treatment room and explained, in his own words, what this process was like for him and how none of it hurt. He jumped right up on the treatment table to show this other child how easy it was and how it all "really wasn't that scary."

The magnitude of emotion I felt that day was unlike anything I had experienced in my career up to that point. I'll never forget the bravery that tiny gentleman displayed for his new friend that day. Being shown and encouraged by his peer that he could do this, too, gave his new friend the courage to start and finish his entire course of treatment. Do not underestimate the power of mentorship through shared experience.

I encourage you to find support in other patients who are experiencing similar treatment. In chapter 3, we discussed asking your social worker about formal support groups available in your area or seeking out support groups online. Additionally, you can ask your radiation oncologist if there is another patient of theirs who would be willing to speak with you regarding their experience.

There are many support groups of all kinds. Please don't underestimate the value of a confidant who can understand exactly how you feel. It can be nice to share similar experiences so you don't have to feel alone—because you aren't. Don't isolate yourself during this time. The validation and support that comes from mentorship in this space is priceless.

Cancer Saved My Life!

I completely understand that this section might not resonate with everyone, and that's okay. This concept might feel snide or callous to hear when you're in the beginning stages of undergoing treatment because the unknown can feel so daunting. However, I would be remiss if I didn't bring up this part of the cancer treatment process.

Early in my career, I had a patient who completed treatment for her breast cancer and returned for a follow-up appointment. She stopped by the treatment machine to visit and thank her team. She said, "This cancer diagnosis was actually the best thing that ever happened to me! I have taken two trips, and I have one more booked—and I've been skydiving! Nothing scares me now!" She continued to tell us she didn't worry so much about the small stuff and had a different, more positive approach to living her life. She credited her cancer diagnosis for "waking up" her life. It was an important lesson I learned in using an unexpected, outwardly negative experience for personal growth and expansion. Talk about turning lemons into lemonade.

This message might seem awfully bold of me to say, and I completely understand this might not resonate with everyone, but I promise you it's not meant to taunt. I'm true to my experience, and this is the truth: I've seen people come out the other side of cancer treatment changed for the better, really making it a point to start *living* their lives. In general, it's not uncommon to hear about life-changing experiences that allow some people to start thinking and living their lives differently. If you choose, you can allow this diagnosis to be that for you, reframing the way you think about your diagnosis.

I implore you to think about what you want your life to look like *after* your treatment. Imagine yourself making it through this and using the experience to *grow yourself stronger*. A cancer diagnosis can be an opportunity to wake up your dormant dreams and start living a life fueled by hope and inspiration for positive changes. Take that dream vacation you always wanted to go on, or visit family that you haven't seen in a while, or mend the relationship with a loved one that has fragmented over the years.

This could be motivating for you if you choose. Let's get you through this unexpected chapter of your life and get back on track to an even more fulfilling and beautiful one! That's the thing about cancer—it can scare you just enough to push you right toward *really* living.

***

Let's take a moment and pause our walk at the shoreline.

Find understanding in the science and support in community.

As you take a deep breath in, recognize how much better you feel now by understanding what's happening to your body when you receive treatment. Some degree of fatigue is inevitable, but you find that truth gives you strength. It's encouraging to have a better idea of what to expect, and this makes you feel that much stronger and ready to move forward.

Exhale as you release the pressure you put on yourself to "do it all." You're human, and you'll face challenges; however, now you have the tools to create a strong and powerful mindset to dispel your self-sabotaging thoughts. Release the heaviness of feeling like no one can understand what you're going through. Now you understand there's another way, and you don't have to carry this all alone.

Take the time you need here to rest. Find yourself slowly reframing your negative thoughts and transforming them to support your own power in your mind. Recognize how good it feels to regain this control.

We find strength together, here in peaceful quiet at the water's edge, as we listen to the waves slowly and repeatedly reach the shoreline. In this moment of rest, I wonder about those glass pieces. Having now grown pitted and softened from their journey through the vastness of the ocean floor, eventually they stumble upon a coral reef. Being gently tossed against the coral by the current of the waves, the edges slowly chip, and their exterior grows that much softer. With their path unpredictable and out of their control, they carry on.

I know transforming your mindset takes effort—and choice. I commend you for your bravery in choosing to walk with me and approach your treatment feeling strong and aware.

We have come so far together, and we still have a little bit more to go. When you're feeling ready, let's walk.

8

Radiation Treatment Side Effects

The Different Causes and What You Can Do about Them

When should I expect the side effects to start?

This is a difficult question to answer with a blanket statement, as everyone's experience with side effects is different. Some people tend to experience side effects around two to three weeks from the start of their radiation. Others might make it through their course of radiation without feeling greatly impacted, then only after completion will they start to feel some side effects.

What are the most common side effects?

The two most common side effects, regardless of what area of the body we're treating, are fatigue and skin irritation. Depending on how many treatments and the type of treatment you're having, the intensity and onset of these side effects will vary greatly. You can speak with your radiation oncologist to help get a better understanding of what side effects you could expect to experience with your tailored radiation treatment.

Fatigue

The Cause

Completing a course of radiation treatment can be a lot to work through physically, emotionally, and mentally. There are many contributing factors at play when considering fatigue in general, as I've mentioned before from a few different angles. We discussed the physical contributor of fatigue in chapter 7, covering the science behind the effects of radiation to your body. To briefly recap, your body will work hard at enacting its natural cell cycle process to repair the damaged cells from the radiation beam. While this makes radiation a highly effective treatment, it also is one of the main reasons why people grow so fatigued during this type of treatment. The subconscious healing process inside your body can be very taxing, especially near the end of your radiation treatment. Not only is your body naturally working hard to heal itself, but your mind also has a whole other set of factors that can intensify your fatigue.

There are multiple contributing factors to consider when discussing mental and emotional fatigue in this space. It's no secret that braving through a cancer diagnosis and treatment is trying, to say the very least. Psychologically navigating your diagnosis and radiation treatment can be complicated. You'll have great days, and you'll have challenging days. The roller coaster of emotions can be exhausting and frustrating. As previously mentioned in chapter 7, integrating the sometimes weeks-long radiation treatment schedule into your already demanding work and family life, all while trying to maintain balance, can be very challenging. The hard truth is that trying to maintain the normalcy of your everyday life and schedule while getting cancer treatment sometimes isn't possible. The frustration that comes from this can often exacerbate the emotional component. With cancer already an unwanted and uninvited part of the equation, the stress is palpable.

You must learn to give yourself grace for persevering through each step of this, from diagnosis to treatment. Even with the science of fatigue out of the equation, juggling the psychological portion alone is enough to cause significant fatigue that can affect your daily habits, interactions, schedule, and mental health. What an understatement to say that this is a lot to have on your plate.

What You Can Do about It

Truly, managing fatigue is very personal and can change day to day depending on how you're feeling. Sometimes the fatigue makes you feel like you want to cancel those dinner plans or sneak in a nap so you can get some much-needed extra rest. Sometimes fatigue can be lessened by getting some fresh air and going for a walk or simply going outside and sitting in a chair.

It's likely your inner circle of family and friends have offered their help to you during this time. Whether it's a meal, dropping off the kids at practice, or giving you a ride to and from your treatment, accept some help. Utilizing offered support doesn't make you weak. In fact, in this instance especially, I believe it makes you stronger and smarter—smart enough to know you're approaching your breaking point of being overwhelmed and stressed, and strong enough to let someone else help support you through it. I bet if the tables were turned, you would likely offer the same help. There's no award for pushing yourself past your limits and continuing to "do it all." Instead, nurture yourself by creating space for your body and mind to heal.

My best advice is to take it day by day and *listen to your body and your mind.* Every day will be different. If you had a rough day on Tuesday, don't let that automatically set you up for discouragement on Wednesday. It's a new day, so let it be new. Try not to set yourself up with the expectation that the same challenges will plague you the next day. When it comes to fatigue, your body needs rest to heal, and your brain needs space to relax and process.

How Long Fatigue Lasts

I would like to be forthright in letting you know this answer can be hard to hear. By now, you understand that each person's treatment is highly individualized, so rest assured everyone's experience with this will be different. There are many factors that impact each person's experience in how quickly they'll regain some of their energy, and, in general, this can take some time.

Even though you've stopped *physically* coming in for radiation treatment, the effects of the radiation are still taking place in your body. (I want to be very clear: there is no radiation *in* your body. It's just the effects of the healing process on the cells that received radiation that I'm referencing here). These effects can last beyond treatment delivery, even though you're no longer physically receiving radiation. In general, people's energy levels can begin to increase around the two-week mark after radiation is complete. Let me emphasize that this is a generalization. Many different factors can impact your energy rebound rate, such as any other treatment or medications you're continuing to receive, how much rest you are able to get, how quickly you jump back into other responsibilities, and so on.

I understand this can be hard to hear, and very frustrating for some, but you *must* acknowledge that your body is working very hard to heal itself, and so it's best for you to be patient. The best thing you can do is to gift yourself this understanding. Your energy levels will get better, but it could take a few weeks to even a month or so before you feel improvements. Know that radiation treatment is a process, and this process takes time. Getting your energy back to where it once was will reveal itself in an increasing fashion.

Skin Irritation

The Cause

Skin irritations occur where the radiation beam enters your body and presents in the shape of the radiation treatment beam. People can experience skin irritations on a wide spectrum that can be greatly influenced by your treatment plan design, the overall radiation dose, and the unique baseline of your skin. These irritations can present like a sunburn, itchy red bumps, blistering, peeling, or dryness of the skin in the treated area.

Depending on your personalized treatment, you might not experience much skin redness at all. If your skin doesn't get red on the outside, don't worry. The radiation is still working *inside* your body.

As you continue with your treatments, it's common to see a distinct outline of darkening skin exactly where the radiation is being directed. Being able to see this delineated outline is a great indicator of a consistently reproducible setup position. So, if you see that outline, you should feel encouraged that everything is very much going according to plan. You can ask your radiation therapists at the beginning of your treatment to show you what area you could expect to see some skin irritation.

What You Can Do about It

It's of utmost importance that you do your best to care for the integrity of your skin in the treated area. The good news is that there are many effective lotions and ointments to help mitigate some of the discomfort you may feel on your skin from the radiation treatment, and the efficacy of each one will depend on the individual needs of each person. There are also new creams and lotions being developed regularly, so feel free to do a little research if you're dissatisfied with the effectiveness of the product you're using. Before applying any new lotion, always check with your team first, as the ingredients will need to be reviewed to ensure this will help your skin and not cause further irritations. Each treatment facility or physician might have preferred lotions for their patients, so it's always best to check with your team before any application of a new lotion.

Tips on Lotion

First and foremost, it's super important to note that whichever lotion you choose should not have any added perfumes, dyes, or aerosols. These can cause extra irritation to your skin where it may already be quite sensitive. Additionally, you'll want to make sure the lotion you've applied is fully absorbed before you come into the room for treatment that day. Having lotion that isn't fully absorbed on top of your skin can make your skin reaction worse (this is easy to avoid, so keep that in mind). Apply your lotion no less than two to four hours prior to treatment (but check this timeline with your treatment team, as each lotion absorption rate can be different). As an aside, you can use any lotion on other areas of your body if the application is not adjacent to or in the area currently receiving radiation treatment.

The Best Overall Lotion and Most Widely Accepted

Aquaphor is a great product. It's the most widely accepted skin treatment for radiation that I have seen patients have success with across the board. It's great for helping with dry or tight skin and is a great lotion to start with right from the beginning of treatment. Make sure, though, not to use the spray version, as the aerosols can be irritating to irradiated skin.

I've seen many patients have success with Aquaphor in the past, but by no means is it the only product out there that can benefit irradiated skin. There are many products available for patients in this space, and I've seen different products used successfully per patient and care-team preference. Regardless of what lotion you choose, I always recommend you double-check with your treatment team to verify its appropriateness before applying.

Important Safety Considerations for Irradiated Skin

When you're receiving radiation treatments, and even once treatments have completed, your skin in the area that received treatment will be *very* sensitive to the sun. Please cover this skin up when you're outside. If you're still under treatment and receive a sunburn in the area we're treating, we might need to delay treatment until your sunburn heals. You really don't want to have an interruption like that for something as avoidable as a sunburn. Keep your skin as healthy as possible while undergoing radiation treatments.

When you're nearing the end of your radiation treatment, skin blistering or peeling can occur, which can create broken skin. It can be difficult to know exactly how to care for your skin at this stage. Your best option is to speak with the nurses at your facility and ask them to show you how to properly bandage this area to avoid causing further skin damage. They'll show you the steps to take to properly care for this delicate skin. In general, you should avoid using silk tape or Band-Aids on top of irradiated skin, as the adhesive is too strong and can cause additional skin peeling when removed. Paper tape (not directly on the irritated part of your skin) that secures loosely placed gauze is a great way to shield your skin from the elements when you're outside of your home.

Hair Loss

The Cause

Hair loss is probably one of the biggest stereotypes surrounding cancer, and we frequently hear concerns about it. Hair loss circumstances are different between radiation treatments and chemotherapy. If you're having radiation treatment only (no chemotherapy), hair loss will occur *only in the places where the radiation beam enters the body*. Therefore, you will not lose the hair on your head if you're receiving radiation to your pelvis (and not having chemotherapy). If you are receiving radiation to your head, brain, or neck area, sometimes hair loss is possible (but remember, only in the small area where the radiation beam *enters* your body). Additionally, if you're having chemotherapy, it's possible for hair loss to occur, but that isn't always the case, as it depends on the drug treatment you're receiving.

What You Can Do about It

There are some treatments available to minimize hair loss with cancer treatment, and the technology surrounding this topic is advancing. At the time of your consultations, you can ask if you should expect any hair loss from your radiation treatment. Furthermore, you can ask your radiation oncologist if you're curious about treatments that might minimize hair loss.

Diarrhea

<u>The Cause</u>

Diarrhea can happen when we're irradiating the pelvis or abdomen because the radiation can irritate the lining of your bowel (both small and large) and can cause food to move through your system a little quicker than you're probably comfortable with. If you're receiving radiation in this area of your body, speak with your team and ask at what point in the treatment you could expect this, if at all, and what they recommend you take to help lessen the severity. Also, it's important to know that continuous diarrhea can cause dehydration, so make sure you're paying extra attention to your fluid intake. I certainly understand the last thing you might feel like doing under these circumstances is drinking more water, but dehydration really does affect all systems of the body, not just your bowels.

<u>What You Can Do about It</u>

The best way to combat diarrhea is with medication. There are a few antidiarrheal products on the market, so you should speak with your nurse to determine which one would be best for you. Additionally, some foods can be irritating to your bowels, so speak with your physician to determine if there are any you should avoid, especially if you're feeling symptomatic.

Dehydration

<u>The Cause</u>

It is very easy to fall into a cycle of dehydration if you're not paying attention to your fluid intake. When you're in the middle of your course of radiation treatments and the fatigue and general unenthused feeling about the process set in, it can be easy to let your nutrition slip. If you're receiving treatment in your mouth, neck, esophagus, or stomach area, sometimes it can be hard to swallow and, therefore, to keep up your nutrition. You might feel uninterested in eating or drinking at times, and that's understandable.

What You Can Do about It

You don't want to neglect your hydration status. Being dehydrated while under treatment can make you feel unnecessarily and overwhelmingly awful, as being dehydrated affects your whole body and all its systems. Drinking water is a simple thing you can do to feel a whole lot better. Support your body as it heals by providing it with hydration so all your systems can work at their optimal level and get you feeling better faster.

Drinking a huge glass of water quickly is not the best way to hydrate comfortably. It's best to work at this in smaller increments. Try setting some goals for yourself throughout the day that feel achievable for you. If you find you're having a very difficult time swallowing and you haven't been able to keep up with your water intake, do yourself a huge favor and bring this to the attention of your team. Don't wait on this or keep it to yourself, because the sooner you tell them, the sooner they can help you with it. Don't wait days on end or for someone to bring it up to you before you mention your challenges. You would be shocked at how much better you feel after we simply get you hydrated properly. Don't sit at home feeling terrible and believing that this is your temporary fate. We're happy to help you through this part, but we need you to work *with us*, so we can get you feeling better relatively quickly.

Nausea

The Cause

Nausea is a very common side effect of radiation therapy treatments. Sometimes nausea can be caused by radiation, and sometimes it can be caused by medications you're taking. Also, some people develop nausea when they're nervous (a common occurrence in the radiation treatment room, as you can imagine). Nausea can affect a wide array of patients receiving radiation, but some of the most common complaints are reported from those receiving radiation to the brain, head and neck, abdomen, and pelvis.

What You Can Do about It

Typically, medication is your best bet for relieving nausea, and an antiemetic from your nurse can do wonders to take the edge off. Some people have luck with ginger as well. If your nausea stems from overwhelming nervousness, an antianxiety medication can sometimes help as well. It's best to speak with your radiation nurse about this so they can help you decide your best course of action.

***

Let's take a moment and pause our walk at the shoreline.

Let's rest.

As you inhale, recognize how good it feels to have a better understanding about side effects and how to manage them. You feel encouraged knowing you have the authority to approach your team with any side effects you experience, no matter how insignificant you think they might be.

As you exhale, release the tension of the anticipatory nerves, because now you know there are tools in place and an entire team ready and willing to help you manage any side effects.

Not knowing what to expect can feel scary. You're courageous for seeking out answers, even if they might be tough to hear. Find peace in your awareness, as this gives you strength to move forward.

Looking out over the ocean in our time of rest, I find tranquility in the smell of freshness in the air and the repetitive cadence of the waves as they meet the shoreline. My mind drifts into a relaxed state, and I am reminded of those glass pieces. Undeniably altered from the currents, the pestering grit from the sand of the ocean floor, and the unrelenting irritation of the salt, each piece faces yet another challenge when waves crash it against the rocks. This unpredictable and unavoidable interaction finds the last bit of unchanged glass and inevitably chips away at those few remaining sharp edges. Having endured these elements with little say or choice, each shard of glass finds itself irrevocably changed.

We're almost finished with our walk—just a little bit more.

9

How We Keep You Safe

The Tools We Use and the Protocols in Place

There are multiple ways we advocate for your safety before beginning treatment, while the treatment beam is actively being delivered, and throughout the entirety of your course of radiation. I'll explain to you the different tools and procedures we have in place to achieve our goal of getting you treated accurately and safely. I'll describe what equipment we use in the head of the linear accelerator to precisely control and direct the radiation beam. You'll learn about the different quality assurance protocols and processes in place to ensure accurate radiation output from the treatment machine as well. You'll discover how we accomplish this and how it all contributes to us delivering radiation treatments confidently. It's my hope that this will bring you peace of mind and help you understand that we take great responsibility surrounding the safety and accuracy of the radiation treatments we deliver.

How We Shape the Radiation Treatment Field

There are a few ways we can shape the radiation field so we can direct *precisely* where we want the radiation to go. Each person's treatment plan could utilize a combination of these different tools.

For therapeutic purposes, the most basic way we shape radiation is by shaping the radiation beam as it leaves the head of the machine and before it touches your body. We do this with *jaws* in the head of the machine where the treatment radiation beam comes out. These jaws can create a rectangle or square that will shape the field of radiation. Sometimes these are the only tools we need to shape the radiation, but often we'll use additional beam-shaping tools to accompany this initial construct to further fine-tune our beam into irregular tumor shapes.

We can refine the shape of the radiation treatment field (in addition to the lead jaws) even further by using tiny lead leaves called *multileaf collimators* (MLC). These tiny lead leaves are supremely effective in precisely shaping the radiation field—even asymmetrical or varied shapes. They can move simultaneously as the treatment machine moves around you to deliver a highly specific, impeccably precise dose. They really are stellar in accomplishing what they're made to do.

Another way we can shape the field of radiation is by an attachment called a *cone* that we put on the head of the machine for a specific type of external beam radiation called *electron*. We place a physical *cutout* that's made from a combination of metals that will block the radiation from reaching your body into this cone and attach it to the head of the machine. The shape of the cutout is what will further help shape the radiation beam before it reaches your body. The shape of this cutout can be custom-made to the shape of your tumor based off of your CT planning scan or utilized in a standard circle, rectangular, or square shape.

It's important to note that the techniques we use today to shape the radiation field are far more advanced than previous decades. Advancements in technology have allowed us to have incredible control over how and where we can direct the beam of radiation. Let this fact bring you comfort, as the treatments have significantly advanced in regards to safety, accuracy, and precision.

How does the department ensure accuracy and precision of the linear accelerator?

In order to ensure the radiation output (the radiation that comes out of the treatment machine) is appropriate for therapeutic treatment, the linear accelerator will consistently go through routine maintenance and quality assurance (QA) checks. There are different checks we run daily, monthly, and yearly to ensure the linear accelerator is behaving appropriately and accurately and precisely producing a high-quality radiation beam. We have QA processes in place to check the machine output, your treatment plan, and the beam delivery in your treatment plan, as well as weekly checks for your chart once your treatment is underway.

There are daily QA checks for the treatment machine that the radiation therapists run before the department opens for treatment each day. These QA checks will confirm the dose consistency and mechanical accuracy of the radiation beam and treatment machine in general. To give you a brief overview of what we check, we make sure the quality of the radiation beam is accurate and precise. We have special equipment we use to check the beam quality—flatness and symmetry of the radiation beam—along with accuracy and precision of all beam-shaping equipment. Additionally, the imaging equipment goes through a QA process to ensure the computers are communicating appropriately and that all imaging systems are functioning properly and accurately.

There are also monthly QA checks performed by the medical physicist, who checks three main things in this QA session: dose dosimetry, machine mechanicals, and imaging quality. Dose dosimetry is in reference to the radiation beam, ensuring that it's of high quality. The machine mechanicals are in reference to the nuts and bolts of the machine—if there are any parts that might need to be replaced or serviced to ensure reliability. Additionally, the imaging components are checked and serviced to ensure high contrast and resolution (factors that contribute to a crisp image for us to use for positioning).

In addition to daily, weekly, and monthly QA, there is an extensive annual QA performed by the medical physicist. This includes the tasks of the monthly QA but also pursues more intensive investigations into the treatment systems and machines, again ensuring high-quality therapeutic beam production.

How does the department ensure accuracy and precision of my personalized treatment plan?

Once your individualized treatment plan has been designed to the satisfaction of the dosimetrist and the radiation oncologist, it then must pass a thorough series of procedural QA checks before your radiation treatment can be delivered to you. Your plan is run through multiple checks by the medical physicist, the dosimetrist, the radiation therapist, and the physician, all of whom must sign off and agree that the treatment plan is accurately delivering the radiation per the radiation oncologist's prescription. Once the plan has been reviewed and approved on paper, the radiation beams are checked by sophisticated equipment used to measure and ensure this plan is delivering the dose appropriately, as intended. Only once the entire QA of your plan on paper and the QA checks of the treatment beams have been approved does the plan become authorized for treatment delivery.

***

We did it! We have completed our walk. Congratulations!

Let's take some well-deserved time here to rest.

Find peace in knowing there is a team behind you and committed to your safety.

Breathe in deeply as you acknowledge how good it feels to have such a comprehensive understanding. Look at how far you've come and how much stronger you are now than when we started our walk. You have choices, and you've chosen to lead with courage and bravery. You feel more confident to pursue treatment than you ever imagined you could. Celebrate this feeling of relief!

As you exhale, tension releases all through your body as you realize you're prepared and well informed. You recognize that the grip of uncertainty has lessened significantly and fear is no longer in control—you are.

You have the tools and the knowledge now to set your mind to meet your goals and to move forward feeling that much more confident.

As we stand here together admiring the vast greatness of the ocean, I think of that glass now. Encounters with the rocks, salt, coral, currents, and sand have given the glass little choice but to accept that it has changed. Over time, nature's elements have evolved that broken bottle. The color of the glass has developed, having grown richer, more complex, and more vibrant than it once was. What once had razor-sharp edges has now softened, and its shape has smoothed. Rewarded by Mother Nature for its trust and patience, the glass is slowly directed toward the light of the shallows from the dark depths of the ocean floor.

Thank you for spending this time with me as we got to walk and talk. I'm so happy we've completed this walk together, but more importantly, you should feel deeply proud of yourself.

Turn around and look at all the steps we've taken together. Even in the moments when your feet sank in the sand and your legs grew tired, you continued to take steps, one in front of the other. Choosing to not let fear take control, you persevered.

Conclusion

Taking those first few steps through your cancer treatment process can leave you feeling alone in the dark abyss, much like shattered glass entering the ocean at the mercy of the waves. What started out as a broken version of itself, tossed into the unknown and unnatural environment of a deep sea, returns to the shoreline as a treasure: sea glass.

Without much choice but to endure the obstacles as it feels out of place in this new environment, the glass eventually leaves the ocean more beautiful than its original form—stronger, and with an extraordinary color only experience can create. People stop in their tracks to admire its uniqueness and wonder about its story.

I couldn't help but draw these similarities as I thought about this cancer treatment process. While I've seen pretty much everyone begin this journey with some level of trepidation, I've seen more people arrive at the end of treatment tired and changed but overwhelmingly proud of what they've accomplished—and relieved for this chapter to be over.

It's an undeniable fact to say that cancer will leave you changed. It can change you physically, and it can change you mentally. I encourage you to lean into your own unique story.

When someone discovers sea glass at the beach, they might pick it up right away and admire it as a treasure. Much like sea glass, your story is your treasure. Once you arrive back at the shoreline having completed your treatment and changed from your experience, *you* are now that treasure.

With your newfound treasure, you have the choice about what you'd like to do with it. When some people find sea glass, they choose to keep it for themselves and cherish it in their own way, displaying it in the privacy of their own home, maybe preferring to keep the treasure for themselves and a few close loved ones.

Other people find sea glass and are inspired to share it with others, switching it from their hand to the hands of friends they encounter along their walk on the beach, admiring its rich uniqueness together. You may decide that you want to share your story with others because you never know who's out there and needs to hear it. What will you do with your newfound treasure?

As you've learned the intricacies of the radiation treatment process throughout our time together, I hope you've arrived at the end of our walk feeling better than you did when we first started. You've made it this far. You're undoubtedly stronger than you think. Give yourself credit, don't be afraid to ask questions, reach out for support, and most importantly, be patient with yourself. You're now moving forward with more strength and courage than you ever imagined possible—believe it!

Embrace and take ownership of your experience and decide what you want your unique narrative to look and sound like. Be that person, and believe deep within yourself that inner strength, trust, and patience will soon lead you to the shoreline as well.

Was This Helpful?

If this book offered you insight, support, or simply made a difference in your day, I'd be so grateful if you shared your thoughts in a review.

Your feedback helps other readers discover the book—and it means the world to authors like me.

Leaving a quick review takes just a minute, and you can do it on Amazon, Goodreads, or wherever you bought the book.

Thank you for reading, and for supporting resources that make a difference.

With gratitude,

Margeaux

Glossary

B

Biopsy:

A medical procedure in which cells or tissue samples are taken from your body to be analyzed microscopically to identify potential disease.

C

CBCT (Cone Beam CT):

This is a low-dose CT image that has been equipped specifically to work directly with the linear accelerator. The image this produces provides us with a three-dimensional picture of the area we're going to be treating in real time, so we can make millimeter adjustments to your positioning and ensure adequate dose coverage for the intended area.

Cell Cycle Process:

A naturally occurring process within your body that refers to a series of events that take place in a cell so it can grow and divide, producing more of the same cell. This natural process takes about two weeks to complete from beginning to end.

Chemotherapy:

The use of drugs to kill microscopic cancer disease throughout your body, which is why this type of treatment is referred to as *systemic*.

Claustrophobia:

Fear of small or enclosed spaces.

CT (Computed Tomography) Scan:

A medical imaging technique that produces three-dimensional images of the inside of the body. Sometimes contrast will be used for this diagnostic scan. Contrast can be administered orally (by mouth) or intravenous injection (by vein), or, not at all. This decision is at the discretion of the physician who ordered the scan. If contrast is injected, it's used to highlight the features of the blood vessels clearly. If contrast is swallowed by mouth, it'll display the features of the digestive tract.

CT Simulation:

The appointment intended for use of a CT scanner to acquire a three-dimensional picture of you in the exact position you'll be in for your treatment. The scan acquired from this appointment will be utilized to design your individualized treatment plan.

Curative Intent:

An overarching treatment goal of a cure.

D

Debulking:

This is the procedure for when the entirety of a tumor cannot be removed with surgery, but they may be able to significantly decrease its size within your body. This type of surgery is an option if your tumor is located near critical or sensitive structures in the body, and the surgeon might not be able to safely access all of it without affecting other systems.

F

Front Desk Administrative Staff:

These staff members will check you in at the front desk each day for your appointment and are usually responsible for guiding you with insurance questions or scheduling additional diagnostic imaging appointments for you, if that has been requested by your physician.

G

Genetic Counselor:

Speaking in the world of oncology specifically, this member of the team will meet with the patient to review the results that the geneticist, pathologist, and biologist provides. They'll be able to help you understand if there is a hereditary link in your genes for your cancer that could be passed down from, or to, your blood relatives.

H

Hormone Therapy:

A type of drug treatment that will slow or stop cancer cells from growing by blocking or lowering the level of hormones in your body that your cancer might use as a food source. This type of treatment only works for cancer types that are hormonally related, such as breast and prostate cancer.

I

Immobilization Device:

Created at the time of CT simulation (and used for each radiation treatment) to stabilize and isolate the area of the body intended to be treated with radiation.

Immunologist:

This member of the team is board certified and responsible for studying how your body's own natural immune system response affects the cancer cells in your body. By understanding the biological connection between your immune system and your cancer, the immunologist provides your oncology team with information that can help determine which drug treatments will be most effective in using your own immune system to help fight your cancer.

Immunotherapy:

A type of drug treatment that can boost or aid your body's own immune system to provide effective support to treat your cancer.

L

Lead Cutouts:

A lead piece of equipment placed into an electron cone and used to shape the radiation field for a specific type of external beam radiation treatment called *electron*.

Lead Jaws:

A component within the head of the linear accelerator responsible for shaping the radiation treatment field into a square or rectangle.

Linear Accelerator:

The machine that delivers therapeutic radiation treatment.

Localized Treatment:

Treatment that's applied to a specific and targeted area.

Medical Dosimetrist:

A board-certified and highly trained individual who understands how different body tissues tolerate radiation. They'll develop and design the optimum treatment plan for you, your body, and your cancer specifically.

Medical Oncologist:

The physician who is responsible for directing and designing your chemotherapy, immunotherapy, and other drug therapy treatments. They'll work closely with your radiation oncologist if it's decided that you'll have systemic drug or chemotherapy treatments in addition to the radiation therapy treatment.

Medical Physicist:

A board-certified team member responsible for the maintenance, upkeep, and operations of the linear accelerator and CT simulator in the department. They oversee all the radiation treatment planning and quality assurance for the linear accelerator as well as individualized treatment plans.

MRI (Magnetic Resonance Imaging):

A diagnostic medical imaging scan that does not use radiation; rather, it uses a combination of radio waves and magnetic fields to create detailed images. This type of imaging is useful for seeing delineation among soft tissues within the body.

MLCs (Multileaf Collimators):

Tiny lead blocks positioned in the head of the linear accelerator that aid the lead jaws in shaping the radiation field. They can move simultaneously as the linear accelerator rotates to deliver treatment and are exceptional in forming irregular shapes for radiation treatment delivery.

N

Nutritionist:

A great resource for any dietary questions or concerns you might have if you're struggling with eating food or significant weight loss due to the radiation treatment. You can meet with them on an as-needed basis or regularly if requested by your oncologists.

O

On-Treatment Visit (OTV):

A weekly appointment that's scheduled during your treatment to briefly meet with your radiation oncologist and nurse to check in or address any concerns. Also referred to as a weekly treatment management (WTM).

P

Palliative Intent:

A treatment goal of pain and symptom relief, not necessarily a cure.

PET (Positron Emission Tomography) Scan:

A medical imaging scan that uses an injectable radioactive chemical (called a *radiotracer*) to visualize areas in the body where there's increased cellular activity.

Positional Imaging:

Images that are taken in the radiation treatment room and used for positional comparison with the image from your treatment plan.

Positive Margins:

These refer to residual cancer cells present in the body after surgery has been completed.

Portal Films:

This type of imaging produces a two-dimensional picture like that of a routine X-ray.

Q

Quality Assurance (QA) Checks:

The different machinery (linear accelerator) checks that we run daily, monthly, and yearly in radiation oncology. Additionally, we have QA checks for process and beam delivery for each treatment plan developed.

R

Radiation Oncologist:

The physician who will be constructing and directing your radiation treatment. They'll work closely in collaboration with surgical and medical oncologists to design a comprehensive cancer treatment plan for you, with their focus specifically on your radiation treatment. They'll decide the total radiation dose you'll receive, how many treatments you'll receive them in, and the daily dose. Once you've started treatment, you'll see them for weekly check-ins alongside your radiation nurse.

Radiation Therapy:

The therapeutic use of a high dose of radiation to treat and kill cancer cells. This kind of treatment is localized—meaning it doesn't go all through your body and will only be delivered to a pinpointed location.

Radiation Nurse:

This nurse works specifically with your radiation physician. They'll help you manage your side effects and will be a great liaison between you and your radiation physician for any questions or concerns. You'll see them for weekly check-ins after your treatment or on an as-needed basis.

Radiation Therapist:

The team member responsible for delivering each radiation treatment.

Radiation Treatment Plan:

The document that outlines the exact area to be treated with radiation, the radiation dose intended for each structure/target, treatment machine angles, and treatment field size and shape.

Radiosensitizer:

A drug that works with therapeutic radiation to make the cells more vulnerable to the treatment radiation.

Researchers:

Staff who work behind the scenes in a radiation department and are responsible for collecting information from patients who want to participate in data collection or new drug studies.

Resimulation:

This is when your treatment team brings you back to the CT scanner to be scanned again. The resimulation might be ordered for tumor shrinking or swelling, as well as position changes for your treatment.

S

SGRT (Surface-Guided Radiation Therapy):

This technology allows us to use the surface of your skin to align your body for treatment and doesn't include the use of radiation to do so.

Social Workers:

A phenomenal resource for social and emotional support. They can inform you about available support groups for patients like yourself, and they're also great listeners.

Support Groups:

A community of people who are facing the same health challenges as yourself and can provide support for you before, during, and after completion of treatment. Some patients have found success with online community support, and some patients prefer to attend support groups that are run locally.

Surgery:

A localized treatment that can be used to physically remove the cancer in your body.

Surgical Oncologist:

This is a surgeon who specializes in oncology. Typically, the techniques, processes, and skill set are more specialized than a general surgeon. They'll work closely with the radiation oncologist to help understand where the cancer is in your body.

Systemic Treatment:

Treatment that goes throughout the entire body.

T

Tattoos:

Permanent ink markings that help the radiation team get you into the correct position for treatment. These tattoos are the size of a very small freckle and often have a slightly blue tint. The tattoo placement isn't necessarily indicative of exactly where the radiation will be delivered; rather, the tattoos aid in the reproducibility of patient positioning by providing a consistent mark for the treatment team.

Treatment Console Area:

This area is directly adjacent to the treatment room and where the radiation therapists sit when they're delivering radiation treatment. There's an audio box and visual monitor in this space, so the radiation therapists can hear and see you the entire time they're delivering treatment.

U

Ultrasound:

A noninvasive diagnostic imaging technique that uses sound waves to create images.

V

Virtual Simulation or V-Sim:

The V-sim appointment is designed as a dry run for your treatment plan. We're checking to ensure that your position is reproducible and everything your physician is intending to treat is in fact lining up appropriately. We utilize imaging to confirm that everything we've planned sets up perfectly. You're ready to start your personalized radiation treatments officially after this appointment.

W

Weekly Treatment Management (WTM):

A weekly appointment that's scheduled during your treatment to briefly meet with your radiation oncologist and nurse to check in or address any concerns. Also referred to as an on-treatment visit (OTV).

Acknowledgements

To Mom, Dad, Alex, and Caroline, how lucky am I to have a team of parents who believe in me as much as you four. Thank you for encouraging me to be courageous, challenge myself, and explore life outside of my comfort zone. You've provided me with every opportunity imaginable. I'm so grateful to you all for your love and support in life and also with this book. I love you all so much!

To Katie, Christiana, and Maddie, three women who have done more for my spirit than anyone. My trusted confidants, support system, and greatest cheerleaders. You have never wavered in lifting me up and believing in me. I couldn't be more grateful. You gals are my rocks, and I love you so much!

To Alisha at Alisha Maria Photography, thank you for sharing your gift and producing the most beautiful photographs to help share my message. I'm blessed to call you my cousin but feel even more fortunate to have you as a confidant and true friend. I'm forever grateful to you for the unwavering encouragement you've shown me both with this book and in our lives together. What a special soul you are to me—I love you so much!

To Maida, what a beautiful and fun friendship our families have shared over the years. You have no idea how much peace of mind you gave me throughout this process. Thank you for your expertise, encouragement, warm conversation, and mentorship. Your support has truly been invaluable to me. Thank you from the bottom of my heart!

To Nouna (Debbie), thank you for being the first person I trusted to read my very first draft. Your guidance and advice in helping me navigate the early stages of this book's development were invaluable. Thank you for your encouragement and teacher's touch. I love you so much!

To Matt and Julie at We Are Almanac, LLC, two beautiful strangers who quickly became trusted confidants. Thank you for believing in me and my message and for fostering a space for me to bloom. This book would not be what it is today without your support, encouragement, and beautiful creativity. Working with you two on this project has been one of my biggest blessings. Thank you from the bottom of my heart!

To my team at Bublish, your guidance and expertise have been invaluable to me. Thank you for believing in my message and for your professionalism. Finding your team has been nothing short of a blessing. Working with you has been so exciting and fun! Without you, I wouldn't have been able to reach all of those who needed to hear what I had to say. Thank you doesn't begin to cover it!